TRACE YOUR
GENES
TO HEALTH

MORE VITAL HEALTH TITLES:

TRACE YOUR
GENES
TO HEALTH

Chris Reading, M.D.
with Ross Meillon

VITAL HEALTH PUBLISHING
Ridgefield, CT

Trace Your Genes to Health: Use Your Family Tree to Guide Your Diet and Enhance Your Immune System

Chris M. Reading
B.Sc., Dip.Ag.Sc., M.B., B.S., F.R.A.N.Z.C.P., F.A.C.N.E.M.
Ross S. Meillon

© C.M. & A.W. Reading
© R.S. & H. Meillon

Second Edition published by Vital Health Publishing, 2002

First published in 1984 by Fontana Australia, Sydney
under the title *Relatively Speaking*
Reprinted 1985
Keats Publishing edition published 1988
under the title *Your Family Tree Connection*
Reprinted 1999

Library of Congress Cataloging-in-Publication Data

    Reading, Chris M.
       Trace Your Genes to Health

       Bibliography: p
       1. Medical genetics 2. Genetic disorders - Complications and
       sequelae
       3. Health status indictors. 4. Food allergy - Complications
       and sequelae
       5. Genealogy.   I. Meillon, Ross S.   II. Title
RB155.R33 1988   616'.042   88-6801
       ISBN 1-890612-23-5

Australian National Library Cataloguing-in-Publication data:

    Meillon, Ross 1936-
       Relatively speaking

       Includes index
       ISBN 0 00 636726 7

       1. Medical genetics - Popular works.
       1. Reading, Chris. 1938-   II. Title
616'.042

Trace Your Genes to Health is not intended as medical advice. Its intent is solely informational and educational. Please consult a health professional should the need for one be indicated.

———————

Dr. Chris Reading graduated in medicine from Sydney University in 1968 and qualified in psychiatry in 1973. He then specialized in organic psychiatry, and subsequently became interested in research into vitamin-mineral deficiencies, metabolic disorders, food allergies and clinical immunology/ecology and genetics as it applies to neuropsychiatric disorders. It was in this area that he became increasingly aware of the medical significance and implications of the family tree.

Dr. Reading is currently in private practice in Sydney. He has published many medical articles on his particular areas of research and interest.

———————

Ross Meillon had many years of experience in the world of advertising, writing everything from press releases to television commercials. He joined here with his brother-in-law, Dr. Reading, to help write *Trace Your Genes to Health*.

To Wendy, Helen, Michael,
Robert, Suzanne, Kim
and Sharon.

Foreword

The good clinician is a detective as was Sherlock Holmes, for each patient presents with a unique set of symptoms and signs. This uniqueness is set within a family, which includes close and distant relatives. The greater the number of genes we share with our family members, the more apt we are to share biochemical and pathological problems. Thus, identical twins are almost certain to share conditions such as depression, manic-depressive psychosis and schizophrenia: much more so than are fraternal twins.

Dr. Chris Reading realized that this principle could be used to help him diagnose and thus treat psychiatric patients more effectively. Physicians are taught to take a family history. This is usually a brief recitation of other members of the family with similar illnesses. Dr. Reading has gone much further. He uses a detailed family pathology tree to help diagnose (i.e., patients are asked to compile the illnesses found in all their relatives). An examination of this tree immediately points to a pattern of illnesses. The patient is a member of this family and is apt to share many of these problems.

A good clinician examines all relevant information. In this book, Chris Reading and Ross Meillon describe how one derives the family tree, how it is used to diagnose and treat, and some of the remarkable recoveries which follow.

When I first read this manuscript over a year ago, I was delighted and impressed with this novel, practical and scientific approach. I promptly urged Dr. Reading to publish this material as soon as possible. At last, here it is. It adds an exciting new dimension to orthomolecular medicine. Further, it is possible to use these family trees to advise families on where they are vulnerable and what to do about it. This is genetic counseling that surpasses any currently being offered at some medical schools.

This first orthomolecular book on genetic sleuthing and treatment will be one of the classics of our time.

Dr. Abram Hoffer, M.D., Ph.D.

Dr. Abram Hoffer, an internationally recognized authority on orthomolecular nutrition, schizophrenia, senility and preventative medicine, is President of both the Canadian Schizophrenia Foundation and the Huxley Institute of Biosocial Research (New York).

Contents

Introduction

For some years now, I have begun my consultations with new patients by making an unusual request. I have asked them to compile their family trees.

No, I'm not a frustrated genealogist. And I'm not trying to find out whether my patients are descended from royalty, common folk or convicts. My purpose is most definitely a medical one – because I have discovered that a family tree can do very much more for you than just tell you who you are and where you've sprung from. It can be a major breakthrough to better health for you and your family. In many cases, it can quite literally make the difference between life and death.

To achieve such a startling result, of course, it has to be a special sort of family tree. It has to contain as much medical information as possible about every person on it. So when I ask people for a family tree, they have to set about speaking to parents, grandparents, aunts, uncles and cousins, to find out as much as they can about the illnesses, aches, pains, symptoms, causes of death, etc., suffered by their relatives and forebearers.

When they can put that kind of data on a family tree, the results are, in most cases, little short of astounding. Such a family tree can reveal the factors that are causing a wide variety of illnesses in your family, and show you how to overcome them. What's more, it can predict who in your family is at risk for which serious illnesses in the future – and do so in time for life-saving preventative action to be taken.

Perhaps most exciting of all, the study of medically detailed family trees can, I believe, throw new light on the causes of such tragic diseases and conditions as cancer, heart attacks, strokes, schizophrenia, dementia, Down's Syndrome, muscular dystrophy and multiple sclerosis. It can even lead to your getting fewer coughs, colds and bouts of flu.

Now, I'm sure that all this sounds, to put it mildly, somewhat controversial. And it is. There are doctors who'll dismiss it as a load of old cod – just as there are doctors who automatically label any form of alternative therapy as quackery. But there are many more doctors around the world who are seeing real and thrilling possibilities in the family tree approach to health. After all, as you'll discover from this book, it's not just a happy little theory I've dreamed up. It's an observation solidly based on the study of actual family trees – more than 2000 of them, at the time of this writing.

When you've seen some of the evidence, I think you'll share my excitement at the healing potential that family trees contain. In this book, we'll see that potential fully realized in many sick peoples' lives. We'll see how their breakthrough to health came from their family trees – sometimes through diagnosis, sometimes through an indicated line of treatment, sometimes through prediction and prevention.

Invariably, the family tree breakthrough came after all conventional medical approaches had failed. After we've digested those thought-provoking cases, I'll show you how to compile your own family tree and fill it with relevant medical information. And to help you interpret it, we'll brush up on some basic genetics.

Then we'll discuss the practical part: how to use your family tree to reduce your risks for a whole host of illnesses, ranging from colds to cancer, heart disease, strokes, psychoses (mental illness) and dementia. We'll also look at the best way of presenting your family tree to your doctor, to help him or her do a far better job of caring for you and your family.

Lastly, we'll examine some exciting family trees that might well be shedding new light on supposedly *incurable* illnesses. And all the way through, we'll see some fascinating family-tree-based evidence suggesting that allergies, especially to grains, may be the basis of many more illnesses than has previously been realized.

We'll see, too, how family trees bring together a lot of the work now being done in various branches of alternative medicine – how they integrate genetics, nutrition, allergies and environmental factors into a unified approach to health and wholeness.

Many of the family trees in this book have real and urgent implications for medical research. When you compile yours, you may well suspect that it does, too. If so, you'll find an address in Chapter 11 where you can send it – so that, ultimately, thousands of other people may benefit from it as well.

Tracing the family tree has become an absorbing hobby, with a vast number of adherents. Now the family tree approach to health gives it significance beyond the thrill of discovering the family's origins. It turns it into an intensely practical venture that not only gives you a sense of identity, but the best possible chance for healing now and ensuring a healthier future.

It could, in fact, save your life.

How did I stumble upon the family tree approach to health? Almost by accident.

About four years ago, a lady we'll call Joanne Woodbridge came to see me. Her problem was manic-depressive illness, and it wasn't hers alone. No fewer than five generations of her family had suffered from it, starting with her great-grandfather and running through to her nephew.

That just had to be more than coincidence. What on earth, I wondered, could produce such a picture? Was there anything else running in her family that might cause it? Suddenly, I thought of asking her to draw up a family tree. She did so. And the mystery was solved.

What did we discover in the Woodbridge family tree? You'll find out in Chapter 4.

Two results flowed from the solution to the Woodbridge mystery. Joanne and her relatives were freed from manic-depressive illness. And I was launched into the investigation of a powerful new tool for diagnosis, treatment and prevention: the family tree.

———————

Since writing the first edition of this book, I have studied many thousands more health family trees. There have been new and exciting developments confirming what I predicted in 1984. For instance, it is now an established fact that cancer cells can and do have receptors not only for hormones in certain cancers but also for food fractions (lectins) literally "feeding the cancer," and these should certainly be removed from the diet of patients with cancer.

This new updated edition discusses some of these new developments in the likely causation of Multiple Sclerosis, Motor Neuron disease, cancer, coronary artery disease, and arthritis such as osteoarthritis, SLE (lupus), scleroderma, Sjogren's Syndrome, synovitis/rheumatoid arthritis, etc.

It also includes additional new appendices listing tests that can be done to help your family doctor to diagnose the causes of hereditary illnesses, thus helping save the lives of your relatives and friends as well as yourself. These appendices contain information useful both to yourself, your relatives and your family doctor and should open up whole new avenues of research into the better diagnosis and treatment of many serious chronic and degenerative diseases, thereby offering new hope for prevention and correction.

Now, read on to see what I've discovered in family trees during the past twenty years – and to see what your family tree can do for you.

PART ONE

How Family Trees
Are Helping People

The proof of the pudding, they say, is in the eating. So, in this first part of the book, we'll look at several case histories and see just how the people involved were helped by their family trees.

Most were people who were very seriously ill indeed. With some, the desperate need was for a diagnosis of a baffling condition. With others, the condition was known, but no one knew how to treat it. With others, again, the problem was to work out whether they were at risk for a serious illness, and, if so, how to prevent it.

In every case, the family tree provided the answer – a diagnosis, a line of treatment, a reassuring prediction or a path to prevention.

We'll also, in this section, digress briefly into some basic genetics, to help us grasp the principles behind the family tree approach to health.

1

How a Family Tree Solved a Mystery

It's not his real name, but let's call him Jack. He was a hard-working professional man in an Australian country town. Besides running a successful practice, he was deeply immersed in the district's activities. Many good causes benefited from his involvement. Deservedly popular and respected, Jack was in every way a leader in his community.

And then he went off the rails.

Normally the most practical of men, he launched with gusto into a highly ambitious project, totally outside his own field. It was obviously going to be a disaster from the word go, and it was. At the same time, irregularities began to creep into his professional practice. They weren't minor ones, either. Large sums of money were involved, and soon both the law and Jack's professional association were knocking on the door.

Just before that happened, Jack's whirlwind round of activities came to an abrupt halt. He collapsed in his office, with symptoms that seemed, at first, to suggest a nervous breakdown. A sharp-eyed doctor at the local hospital examined Jack closely. He saw two things that pointed to a more serious diagnosis: slight paralysis of the left side of the face and some loss of function in the left hand. An ominous combination.

Jack was immediately flown to Sydney for special tests. These, the doctor believed, would confirm the sad diagnosis: a brain tumor would explain both the physical symptoms and Jack's out-of-character behavior.

However, neither brain scans nor x-rays found the slightest trace of a tumor. So the nervous-breakdown theory was resurrected. But it didn't quite fit either the

3

physical symptoms or the bizarre behavior which, investigation showed, had been building up for some time. What was going on in Jack's life?

The hospital psychiatrist was called in. He tackled the problem along classic Freudian lines, looking for clues somewhere between Jack's childhood experiences and his current sex life. He labeled the problem *hysterical amnesia*, but could offer no useful advice on treatment.

At that point, Jack was referred to me.

When I first heard a summary of the symptoms, I thought Jack would prove to be schizophrenic. But as I talked with him, I changed my mind. There was none of the rigidity or faltering grasp of reality that usually accompany schizophrenia. I found Jack extremely intelligent, likeable and as puzzled as anyone else by what was happening to him. He had absolutely no memory of the strange things he had done. He was understandably depressed and worried, a little confused, and very tired.

So, I adopted the tack I have taken for several years – the one which invariably makes new patients blink in astonishment. I asked Jack for a family tree: for as detailed a family tree as he could provide, with special reference to his forebears' medical problems and causes of death, for as far back as he could go. It took a few days, as it normally does. But with the help of his mother and other relatives, Jack put together a pretty good family tree, with quite a bit of solid medical information.

And there, staring me in the face, was the answer. Jack's maternal grandmother, great uncle, great aunt and mother had all had conditions suggesting marked allergies to grains. The country town where Jack had moved only a few years earlier, after a lifetime in Sydney, was in the heart of a wheat-growing area. For certain periods of the year, the air was thick with wheat dust.

Immediately, I ran Jack through detailed allergy tests. I knew what I would find, and I wasn't disappointed. He had a massive allergy to grains, including wheat and wheat dust. He couldn't have chosen a worse place to live.

Jack was suffering from allergic encephalitis, a serious inflammation of the brain, brought about by his allergic reactions to wheat dust and grain. That was more than enough to account for his physical symptoms and apparent personality change.

From then on, it was plain sailing. I put Jack on a grain-free diet, pumped a lot of relevant vitamins into him, and forbid him to go anywhere near the wheat belt – even to pack up his belongings. His improvement was rapid and lasting. Within weeks, virtually all his symptoms disappeared. Four years later, he feels better than he has ever felt in his entire life.

THE FAMILY-TREE WAY TO BETTER HEALTH

The moral of Jack's story is my reason for writing this book. I am convinced that many, if not most, of the ills that beset us can be diagnosed, predicted – and often prevented – by studying our family trees. Such a study can, I believe, tell you why particular illnesses are occurring in your family. It can provide otherwise unobtainable clues to diagnosis and treatment. It can predict who in your family is at risk for certain illnesses, and usually enable you to prevent those illnesses, years before they strike. What's more, I'm not just talking about "running-in-the-family" things like asthma and diabetes. I am talking about the very nasty ones: cancer, schizophrenia, heart disease, manic-depressive illness, dementia and pernicious anemia, to name a few.

Am I really claiming that clues to the prediction, prevention and cure of such frightening illnesses can be found in our family trees?

Yes, I am. And even if none of our ancestors has actually had those illnesses, there may still be clues in our family trees as to whether or not we, or our children, are likely to be victims. In other words, I'm saying that many

of the worst diseases from which we suffer are, very frequently, transmitted genetically. Or, more precisely, that
the factors that make us vulnerable to them are passed on
to us from our forebears. That immediately suggests two
very important conclusions.

First, an accurate, detailed family tree is one of the
best insurance policies you can have against illnesses, for
yourself and your children. Why? Because it can tell you
why you're suffering from particular illnesses, and what
to do about them. Furthermore, it can tell you the illnesses that you especially need to watch out for in the
future. For if you know that, you can, in almost every
case, take positive steps to prevent them. I'll elaborate on
that later in the book.

Second, if enough family trees became available for
study, we could identify the genetic factors involved in
the transmission of diseases like cancer and schizophrenia. Such a major breakthrough could finally solve the
mysteries of these illnesses, and lead to effective new
ways of preventing and treating them.

So, I want to encourage you and your family to draw
up as complete and detailed a family tree as possible –
and to do it now, while vitally important older relatives
are still alive and clear headed. If you do, you and your
family will certainly benefit. It could even save a life
within your family circle, and I'm not being overdramat-
ic when I say that. In addition, it could be of tremendous
benefit to all mankind because, lurking in the branches of
your family tree, there could be some vital clues that will
deepen our understanding of a deadly illness.

Please join with me and be a coworker in this genetic research. It's not hard. It's a lot of fun. And there's a
real thrill in finding out more about your family history.
Almost certainly you've got some fascinating characters
back there, hiding in the shadows of time – people
whose genes are in your body now, having helped to
shape you physically, mentally, emotionally and socially.

When you find out more about your background, your own identity grows. You see yourself as part of a historical process, get a deeper insight into who you really are, and see yourself as belonging to an identifiable group of people. You start to understand why *Roots* had such enormous appeal all over the world.

But how do you draw up a family health tree? What should you put on it? Where do you get the information? How can it help safeguard your family's health, now and in the future? How can you use it to help mankind?

This book gives you the answers.

❧2❧

A Crash Course in Genetics

The most remarkable thing about your family tree is that it produced you – a unique human being. Since the world began, no one else has ever had your exact genetic make-up (unless you're one of identical twins, triplets, quads, etc., in which case, you're part of a unique pair or group).

Your story began when a sperm from your father penetrated an egg from your mother, deep in your mother's body. At that miraculous moment, both sperm and egg released 23 tiny particles of living matter, called chromosomes. Each chromosome from the sperm found a matching partner from the egg. They came together – and the first cell of your body was created.

As soon as that single cell existed, your blueprint was finalized. Your physical appearance – potential height, build, facial features, hair color, eye color – was fully determined. Your sex was established. Your latent talents and abilities were laid down. Much of your mental and emotional makeup was decided.

And the potential for various illnesses, some trivial, some serious, was programmed into your being.

How your sex was established

Your sex was established in a particularly interesting way. When I said that each chromosome from sperm and egg found a matching partner, I mightn't have been completely accurate. Of the 23 chromosomes from each side, 22 certainly did find an identical partner. But the other two were the sex chromosomes, one from dad, one from mom. And they may or may not have formed a matching pair. If they did, you're a female. If they didn't, you're a male.

That's because there are two different kinds of sex chromosomes – logical enough in a species divided, as

8

you've doubtless noticed, into two sexes. The two kinds are known as *X* and *Y* chromosomes. The sex chromosome from the mother's egg is always an X variety. But the one from the father's sperm can be either X or Y. And the baby's sex depends on whether an X-type or Y-type sperm wins through to fertilize the egg.

There's an incredible competition among the sperms to achieve that particular honor. At the moment of ejaculation, the man releases a huge number of sperms – from 50 million to 500 million, on the average – into the woman's body. Of those sperms, almost exactly half carry an X chromosome. The other half carry a Y. But only one out of all those millions will enter the mother's egg and fertilize it. The instant that the victorious sperm enters the egg, a chemical process dramatically hardens the egg's covering. All the other sperms are locked out. Immediately, the die is cast. Probably the most important single factor affecting the baby's future has been determined, once and for all.

If the winning sperm is an X-type, its X chromosome will join with the mother's X chromosome to make the new baby a girl. If it carries a Y chromosome, the combination of that and the mother's X will make the baby a boy. Quite possibly, you know all that already. But not everyone does, and, as we'll see shortly, it's important to have the role of sex chromosomes clearly in our minds when we consider how diseases are transmitted genetically.

The sex chromosomes are so named because they determine our sex. The other 22 pairs of chromosomes, the nonsex ones, are known as autosomes. That's another term we'll need to remember, to help us understand the genetic transmission of disease.

GENES: OUR BODIES' BUILDING BLOCKS

How can a mere 46 chromosomes carry the unbelievable amount of information required to create something as complex as you? To answer that, we need to take a very close look at the chromosomes. Under a microscope, they look like tiny threads of jelly (*Figure 1*). Their shapes have reminded various people of worms, crosses, bits of seaweed, knucklebones or pairs of pliers. But if we could see them even more closely (*Figure 2*), we would notice something else again.

Each chromosome is composed of hundreds of little blobs, arranged in line like pearls on a string. The little blobs are called genes, and it is these genes that have made you what you are. Every detail of your physical makeup, and the way your body chemistry operates, is determined by your genes, which have come down to you in an un-broken line from the dawn of human history.

When your earliest ancestor first stood upright and surveyed the world from the edge of the primeval forest,

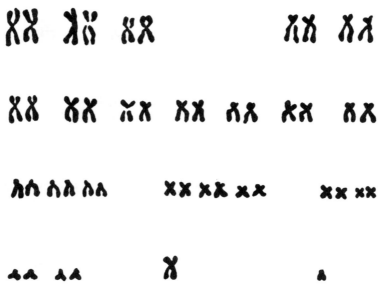

FIGURE 1: the chromosomes

Shapes that remind people of worms, crosses, bits of seaweed, knucklebones or pairs of pliers. Normally, people have 46 identical sets in every cell.

he carried in his body some of the actual genes that are in your body now.

In a book like this, we can only touch very briefly on these incredible building blocks. Basically, however, genes are protein molecules. Their main constituent is a chemical compound called deoxyribonucleic acid, which is generally known by its shortened name of DNA. It is the DNA that gives genes their two most vital abilities: the ability to reproduce themselves, and the ability to produce proteins – the organic compounds that are essential to tissue growth.

There are tens of thousands of different types of human genes. Exactly how many is still uncertain, but most experts put the total number of genes in our 46 chromosomes somewhere round about 100,000.

The truly awesome thing is that each of those genes is different. Each one has a different chemical effect, which is why our bodies develop into organisms of such stunning complexity.

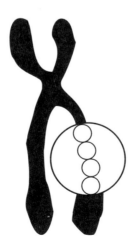

FIGURE 2: **close-up of a chromosome**
Each chromosome consists of multitudes of genes, arranged in line like pearls on a string.

The gene-directed process of development goes into action from the moment of conception. As we have seen, the chromosomes from sperm and egg pair off, and the body's first cell is formed (*Figure 3*). Then each gene creates a replica of itself. As the genes are linked together into chromosomes, that means that each of the 46 chromosomes now has an identical twin standing beside it.

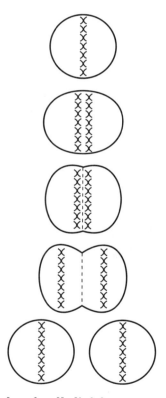

FIGURE 3: the miracle of cell division

From top to bottom: After conception, the first cell has its full complement of 46 chromosomes; each gene then creates an exact replica of itself, so that every chromosome has an identical twin beside it; the two groups of chromosomes move apart; a wall forms between them; the single cell becomes two.

Once that duplication is completed, the newly formed chromosomes move away from their parents. A wall forms between the two groups; the single cell has become two. With unbelievable speed, the process continues. The two cells divide again, into four. The four become eight. The eight become sixteen – and so on, until the baby is complete, ready to be born, with about 26 trillion cells in his or her body.

Every one of those cells has exactly the same set of chromosomes, carrying exactly the same genes, as were in the very first cell. But the cells themselves are as different as they could be. There are skin cells, brain cells, bone cells and hordes of others – all perfectly adapted to their particular roles in an infinite variety of tasks.

How can cells containing an identical set of genes and chromosomes be so different? That's where the different chemical effect of every single gene comes in. As the cell-dividing process continues, some clusters of cells are directed by certain genes to form themselves into internal organs. Some are influenced to mass together to become bones. Others are instructed to spread out horizontally to form skin layers. Between them, all the genes carry the blueprint for a complete human being, and with fantastic precision that blueprint is translated into reality.

Occasionally, however, as with any process on this earth, natural or man-made things go wrong.

CHROMOSOMAL ABNORMALITIES

Sometimes people are born with more than 46 chromosomes in each cell. Sufferers from mongolism, or Down's Syndrome, as doctors call it, are in this category. They have 47 chromosomes in every cell. That might seem a small departure from the normal – especially as the extra chromosome, an autosome, is one of the smallest – yet its physical and mental effects are far-reaching and profound.

Some other conditions also involve an extra chromosome. Men with the Klinefelter Syndrome have an additional X chromosome, which gives them a sex chromosome constitution of XXY. They have underdeveloped sex organs, tend to be mentally retarded and have a higher than normal rate of depression, schizophrenia and other mental and emotional problems.

On the other hand, some conditions come from having fewer than 46 chromosomes. The Turner Syndrome, which affects women, is one. Sufferers have only 45 chromosomes in each cell, the missing one being an X chromosome. Consequently, their sex-chromosome constitution is just simply X, or, as some experts call it, XO. Typically, women with the Turner Syndrome are short, with broad chests and an extra fold of skin on the sides of their necks. They tend to suffer from heart trouble, and are usually mentally retarded.

Many other chromosomal abnormalities have been found in the last few years. As with Down's Syndrome, some of these have an extra autosome, but in a different set of autosomes from the one involved in Down's Syndrome. Several other abnormal sex-chromosome constitutions have also turned up, including XXX, XXXY, XXXXY, XXYY and XXXX.

Knowledge of these aberrations is quite recent. It was as late as 1959 before anyone realized that chromosomal abnormalities cause some diseases. Indeed, the basic fact that our normal chromosome count is 46 was fully established only in 1956. Until then, it had been thought that humans had 48 chromosomes, the same as gorillas, chimpanzees and orangutans. Most conditions, caused by chromosomal abnormalities are obvious and dramatic. Moreover, the people suffering from them rarely have children, and so the conditions are not usually passed on in any direct sense. It's quite different with problems stemming back to rogue genes – what this book is all about.

WHEN GENES TURN TRAITOR

The hereditary nature of such conditions is, very frequently, subtle and hard to detect. As a result, the problem can slip silently through a family for generations, affecting this member, avoiding that one, in an apparently random pattern. It might be a minor nuisance, like premature baldness. It might be a vicious killer, like bowel cancer. But whatever it is, it does leave a genetic trail. Its mode of transmission can be detected, its appearance can be predicted and, in many cases, positive steps can be taken to ward off the effects.

If genes are the building blocks of our bodies, how and why do they sometimes turn traitor and work against us? In broad terms, the answer seems to be that, every now and again, some genes mutate and change their nature. What causes the mutation is largely a mystery. Naturally occurring ionizing radiation is one factor, but only a small one. Man-made radiation and some chemicals are also known to be culprits. However, as gene mutation has been going on ever since human beings first trod the earth, the main causes are obviously natural and yet to be discovered.

A mutation may spring up, run through several generations of a family and then die out when the last person carrying it doesn't have children. Or, the gene may mutate again and lose its capacity to produce trouble. And because gene mutation is occurring all the time, it is just as likely to bob up spontaneously in your generation, as it was to occur back along the time trail trodden by your ancestors. In other words, your future descendants may one day trace the family's genetic misfortunes back to you, and be able then to protect their descendants from whatever your genes started!

The effects of a rogue gene fall into two categories: those that are present at birth (such as color blindness or an extra finger) and those that appear later in life (such as some cancers and psychoses). The errant gene is passed on in any one of a number of different ways, depending on the chromosome on which it is located.

How it is being passed on is far from an academic point. In fact, you have to know how a condition is being transmitted, before you can predict who in the family is at risk for it.

DOMINANT AND RECESSIVE TRANSMISSION

There are six different ways in which a genetic condition can be passed on. The geneticists call them autosomal dominant, autosomal recessive, X-linked dominant, X-linked recessive, X-linked intermediate and Y-linked.

They are not as hard to understand as the names might imply. But before looking at each one in detail, we

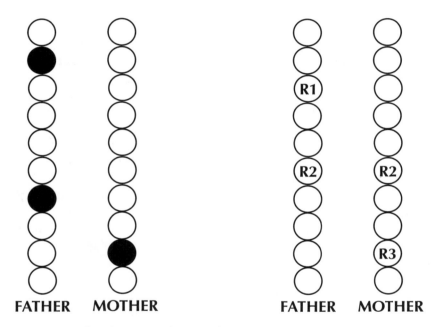

FATHER   MOTHER   FATHER   MOTHER

FIGURE 4: dominant and recessive genes
These diagrams represent the father's and mother's chromosomes about to find their matching partners as they create the body's first cell. In the left-hand diagram, the dominant genes (in black) will *dominate* the genes opposite them, and cause whatever conditions they are carrying to appear in the child. In the right-hand diagram, two recessive genes (marked "R2") are opposite each other on the matching chromosomes. The condition they are carrying will also appear in the child. Those marked "R1" and "R3," however, have no corresponding recessive genes opposite them. Consequently, the conditions they are carrying will not appear in the child.

need to understand what the terms *dominant* and *recessive* mean.

A *dominant* gene is one that acts on its own to produce the particular condition. It "dominates" the normal gene opposite it on the matching chromosome (*Figure 4*), and so its effects can appear even when it is transmitted by just one parent. Like a dominant person, a dominant gene throws its weight around, makes its presence felt, and usually gets its own way.

A *recessive* gene, however, produces the condition only when a matching recessive gene from the other parent is transmitted along with it. In such a case, a double dose of the faulty gene, one from each parent, is needed before the condition can appear.

It doesn't automatically follow that a dominant gene will produce its effect every time. Sometimes, it has what is called a lower *expressivity*, which simply means that, although dominant, it does not always express itself. While one child getting the gene might show the condition, another might escape it altogether, or show it only to a minor degree.

Armed with that information, we can now take an intelligent look at each type of transmission.

AUTOSOMAL DOMINANT TRANSMISSION

Autosomal dominant transmission occurs when there is a faulty dominant gene on one of the autosomes – that is, the nonsex chromosomes – of one parent. And when a parent transmits a faulty gene in an autosomal dominant way, half the children, on the average, boys and girls alike, are at risk for getting it – and with it, whatever defect it is carrying. The operative phrase there is "on the average." Sometimes all the children will get the troublesome gene. Sometimes, none of them will, or maybe one or two. So, on the average, the risk factor is 50 percent.

That's because the faulty gene sits on a chromosome opposite a normal gene on the matching chromosome. And as you will remember, we have 46 chromosomes in

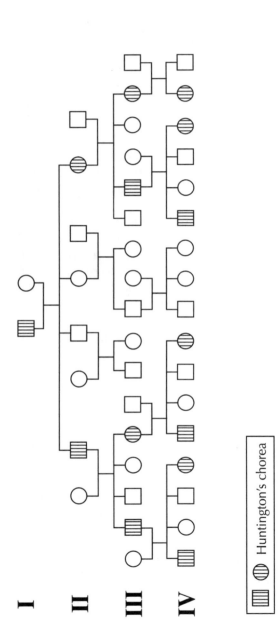

FIGURE 5: autosomal dominant transmission
Because of its autosomal dominant nature, a condition like Huntington's chorea, a terrible mental illness, appears in about 50% of the children, male or female, of those who have it. The children of those who miss it, however, are perfectly safe.

⊕ Huntington's chorea

23 matching pairs in each of our cells. But our germ cells (our sperm or eggs, depending on our sex) have only 23 chromosomes, one from each matching pair. It's pure chance which chromosome from each pair gets into a particular germ cell.

On the average, over your reproductive life, half of your germ cells will get the first chromosome from a matching pair. The other half will get the second one. It's like tossing a coin lots of times – you tend to get half heads and half tails. So, if you have a faulty dominant gene on one of the chromosomes in a pair, you can expect to get it in the half of the germ cells you produce. Which means, on average, that half of your children will get it too.

Figure 5 shows what a family tree looks like when an autosomal dominant condition is running through it. This is typical of the family trees produced by Huntington's chorea, a terrible form of mental illness. It's long been known that Huntington's chorea is transmitted in an autosomal dominant way. It strikes in later life, usually well after a person has had children – and has thus, unknowingly, already transmitted the disease to the next generation.

Notice from this family tree how the condition is passed on relentlessly to about 50 percent of the children of those who have it. The people who missed it don't pass it on, because they didn't get the gene responsible for it. You can see that the children of the sufferers in the present generation would be very much at risk for this terrifying disease. But there would be no way of knowing, in early life, which of them would actually get it. And unfortunately, with Huntington's chorea, not much could be done to protect them from it.

But with many, if not most, conditions, when the risk is so obvious years in advance, there are steps that can be taken to protect people from the disease, or at least to minimize its effects. I'll later be expanding on that theme in considerable detail.

AUTOSOMAL RECESSIVE TRANSMISSION

The second form of transmission, autosomal recessive, occurs when a parent has a faulty recessive gene on one autosome of a matching pair. The effects are not nearly as inevitable as those caused by autosomal dominant transmission – but under the right circumstances, they can be just as severe. As you will remember, a recessive gene does not, by itself, cause the condition it is carrying to appear in the child. Another recessive gene from the other parent, carrying the same defect, must land opposite it on the matching chromosome before its effects will show up.

On the face of it, that would seem to be a pretty unlikely chance. Unfortunately, however, recessive genes are very common among the population at large, and the chances of two coming together are not really remote. Indeed, it has been estimated that each of us carries perhaps three recessive genes capable of causing serious problems in our children, if any of them met up with a similar one from our partner.

Autosomal recessive transmission can, by its very nature, be extremely hard to detect. The recessive gene can glide quietly through generation after generation, giving no hint of its presence. The people carrying it will pass it on to half of their offspring, but neither donors nor receivers will be aware of it. Then one day, the recessive gene will meet its partner and come striding out of the wings to flaunt its effects on center stage.

Those effects can be very diverse, ranging from things like cleft palate and albinism to even more serious conditions, such as cystic fibrosis and adrenal gland cancer. Mild or severe, they will appear, on the average, in 25 percent of the children of a couple who both carry a similar recessive gene. That figure of 25 percent is not hard to understand. We have already seen that, if one parent has a faulty gene, it turns up in half of the germ cells he or she produces. So each child has one chance in two of getting it. But if both parents have a matching faulty gene, the child's chance of getting it from both sides are half those of getting it from one parent alone – that is, one chance in four, or a 25 percent risk factor.

On the average, therefore, faulty recessive genes will hit only half as many children in a family as a faulty dominant gene will. And even when someone does get a double dose of a recessive gene, and picks up whatever condition is being carried, the guilty genes still stay recessive. The person won't pass the condition on, unless his or her partner also happens to have the same recessive gene.

That, of course, is why marriages between cousins carry a higher genetic risk than other marriages. When someone with a trouble-making recessive gene marries a first cousin, the chances are one in eight that the cousin will also have the same gene. Why one in eight? Well, let's imagine that the husband is married to his mother's brother's daughter. There's a 50 percent chance that the husband got his offending recessive gene from his

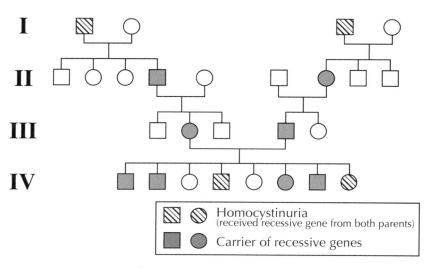

FIGURE 6: autosomal recessive transmission
An autosomal recessive condition such as homocystinuria only appears if both parents carry recessive genes for it. Generation IV shows the typical situation in such a family: 25% have the illness, 25% are normal, 50% become carriers of the recessive gene.

mother. And if she had it, there's a 50 percent chance that her brother (the wife's father) had it too. If he did, he had a 50 percent chance of passing it on to his daughter (the wife). So the chance of husband and wife having the same recessive gene is 50% x 50% x 50% – or .5 x .5 x .5. That works out to one chance in eight – a lot higher than the chance of unrelated husbands and wives having the same recessive gene, which has been roughly estimated at one in a hundred.

It doesn't follow, of course, that cousins can't have perfectly healthy children. In seven out of eight cases, they will. But they do run a higher risk than others of matching their faulty recessive genes, the presence of which might be totally unsuspected.

Naturally, if conditions caused by recessive genes are known to be running in the family, then cousins – or, indeed, any blood relatives – should weigh the odds very carefully before they marry and have children.

A family tree with an autosomal recessive condition, in this case homocystinuria (which we'll meet again later in the book), is shown in *Figure 6*. You can see how the recessive genes have sailed along harmlessly on both sides of the family until they collided. Having wrought their effects, they will return to slinking along in the shadows until they again meet similar genes, or mutate back into a harmless form, or vanish unlamented when their last carrier doesn't have children.

"But," you well may ask, "if recessive genes don't have any outward effects on their own, how can you tell who carried them in previous generations?" That's a good question. The answer is that you tell by deductive means, by working along the links between the people who have the condition.

For example, in generation IV, two people have it. Therefore, their parents must both be carriers. Two generations ago, the father's maternal grandfather and the mother's paternal grandfather were sufferers. Therefore, the father's mother and the mother's father must also have been carriers. And so on.

Note, too, that half the people in generation IV are carriers, while 25 percent dodged the gene altogether. In real life, you couldn't tell initially who was who. Even those carrying the gene won't get homocystinuria, nor will their children. But, if they marry people who do have homocystinuria, or have it running in their families, then the children's chances of getting it would be considerably above average. In other words, everyone in generation IV would be well advised not to marry into homocystinuria families – even though two of them would be perfectly safe in doing so.

The problem is knowing who the two safe ones are. It's easy to look back and see the carriers. To look ahead and see them is, unfortunately, usually impossible.

PROBLEMS ON THE X CHROMOSOME

In both autosomal dominant and autosomal recessive transmissions, sons and daughters are equally at risk, regardless of whether the faulty gene comes from dad or mom. That's not the case with the so-called *X-linked* forms of transmission, to which we will now turn our attention.

As the name implies, X-linked transmission occurs when the problem gene is located on the X chromosome. It has one distinctive feature: Sons are perfectly safe from their father's X-linked conditions, for the simple reason that sons never get their father's X chromosome. They get his Y chromosome, and their X chromosome comes from their mother. However, that certainly doesn't protect males from getting X-linked conditions. Fathers pass them on to their daughters, who pass them on to their sons. So while a man's sons aren't at risk for his X-linked problems, his grandsons are, via his daughters.

X-linked conditions are broken down into three categories: dominant, recessive and intermediate. We'll look at each one in turn.

X-LINKED DOMINANT TRANSMISSION

When the faulty gene on the X-chromosome is a dominant one, the transmission becomes X-linked dominant. It results in a very characteristic family tree, of which *Figure 7* is a typical example.

The condition running through this family tree is manic-depressive illness (which isn't always X-linked, but is in this particular family). See how it's being passed on by the males to all of their daughters, but to none of their sons. The daughters, however, pass it on to an average of half of their children, sons and daughters alike. Because the gene is dominant, its effects appear in virtually everyone who gets it.

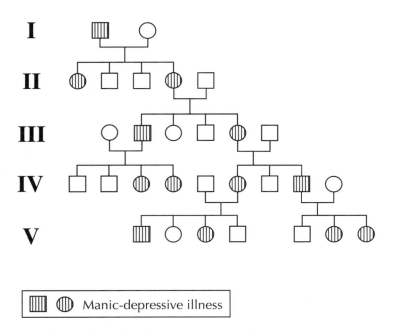

IIII Ⓜ Manic-depressive illness

FIGURE 7: X-linked dominant transmission
Men with an X-linked dominant condition give it to all of their daughters but none of their sons. The affected daughters pass it on to an average of half their children, sons and daughters alike.

This family tree is also a good example of how you can tell which of the unborn children in the next generation are at risk. Just look at the people in the current generation (bottom line) who have the manic-depressive illness. All the daughters, but none of the sons, of the affected male will get it, while all of the children of the affected females will be at risk. The children of those in this generation who escaped the condition will, however, be quite safe.

It's very unlikely, of course, that all those in the next generation, at risk through their mothers, will actually get the manic-depressive illness. As we have already seen, about 50 percent of them will. Unfortunately, there's usually no precise way of knowing which 50 percent – although, for some conditions, predictive tests are now becoming possible.

X-LINKED RECESSIVE TRANSMISSION

The second form of X-linked transmission is X-linked recessive. This is sparked off by a faulty recessive gene on the X-chromosome.

There's a very important difference between X-linked recessive and X-linked dominant transmission. In the dominant version, you will recall, daughters invariably get the condition being carried on their father's faulty gene. But in X-linked recessive transmission, they don't get it – unless their mother happens to have the same recessive gene. Normally, the daughters just become carriers of the father's recessive gene. But when the daughters have sons, a fascinating thing happens – even though the gene is recessive, the sons who receive it will almost always get whatever condition it is carrying.

How can that happen? Didn't we learn earlier that a recessive gene doesn't show its effects unless it meets a matching recessive gene? Yes, we did. And we also learned the reason: The recessive gene's effects are blocked by the normal gene opposite it on the matching chromosome.

However, in the case of the X chromosome in males, there isn't a matching chromosome. The X chromosome, passed on from the mother, is on its own. So there is no normal gene opposite the faulty one to block its effects and, consequently, the effects appear. The son's get the condition for which mom is an X-linked carrier, even though the gene is recessive.

The daughters, on the other hand, are much better off. They also get the mother's X-chromosome with its faulty recessive gene, but they get dad's X-chromosome as well. The normal gene on dad's compensates for the faulty recessive gene on mom's so the girls don't get mom's X-linked recessive condition – unless dad happens to carry the same recessive gene. This is one situation in which girls are on a much sounder genetic foundation than boys.

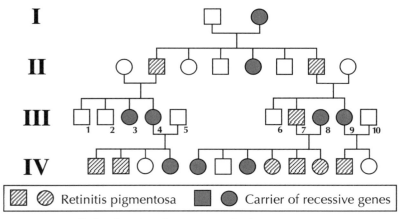

FIGURE 8: X-linked recessive transmission

When a woman carrier of an X-linked recessive condition passes the faulty gene to her sons, the sons always get the condition because there is no matching X chromosome with a normal gene to block the faulty gene's effects. In the next generation, half the daughters of affected sons become carriers, but the son's sons are safe. Note that the carrier females don't get the disorder unless their mother (a carrier) marries a man who has the condition (see people 7 and 8 in generation III). Of their four daughters, two (on average) will be carriers and two will actually get the condition. Those girls who get it will give it to all their sons, and all their daughters will be carriers.

You can see the typical X-linked recessive pattern running through the family tree in *Figure 8*. The condition in this one is retinitis pigmentosa (an eye condition that can lead to blindness). Notice how the girls are carriers; half their sons get it and half their daughters become carriers. Of the sons who get it, all of their daughters become carriers, and their sons miss it.

Once again, it's obvious who needs to watch out for the retinitis pigmentosa in the next generation.

X-LINKED INTERMEDIATE TRANSMISSION

The third form of X-linked transmission, X-linked intermediate, is a sort of cross between the first two. It's really a form of X-linked dominant transmission, in which the dominant gene has a lower than usual incidence of expression. With X-linked dominant transmission, you'll remember, the daughters of an affected man invariably get his X-linked condition. With X-linked recessive, they become carriers. And in both cases, their sons are sitting

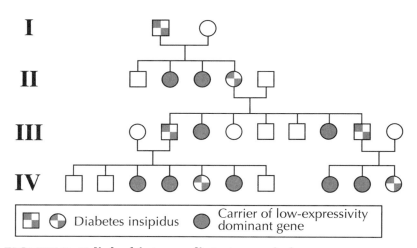

FIGURE 9: X-linked intermediate transmission

If the X-linked condition is *intermediate* in transmission, fewer than 50% of the daughters of affected men get it. The same pattern of risk as in X-linked dominant transmission applies, however, to both sexes in the next generation.

ducks for whatever the problem is. X-linked intermediate transmission produces results that are somewhere in the middle. Some of the daughters get the condition severely. Some get it mildly. Lots don't get it at all. But, once again, the sons are all at risk for it.

Figure 9 shows an X-linked intermediate family tree, with diabetes insipidus (nephrogenic) running through it. At first glance, this could be an X-linked dominant family tree; but a closer examination shows that the number of daughters getting the diabetes insipidus is well below 50 percent. The pattern of risk for both sexes in the next generation, however, is identical to an X-linked dominant situation.

Y-LINKED TRANSMISSION

All in all, the poor old X chromosome seems to carry more than its share of genetic troublemakers. But what

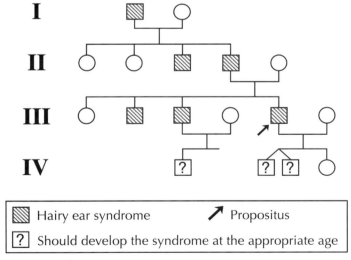

| Hairy ear syndrome | Propositus |

| ? Should develop the syndrome at the appropriate age |

FIGURE 10: Y-linked transmission

Y-linked conditions would always have a father-to-son transmission pattern. So far, only one condition – the hairy ear syndrome – is under strong suspicion of being Y-linked.

about its masculine counterpart? How often does the Y chromosome visit afflictions upon sons and their sons? Surprisingly enough, not very often. Or maybe it's not so surprising when you take a close look at the Y chromosome. It's a very small beastie indeed – much smaller than the X chromosome and most of the autosomes.

Consequently, it carries far fewer genes than the X-chromosome, which means far fewer genes to mutate and cause trouble. And that, without doubt, is something to gladden the hearts of male chauvinists the world over.

In fact, only one condition so far is under strong suspicion of being Y-linked. And it's a harmless enough one: the tufts of hair that some men have sprouting out of their ears. Geneticists are divided as to whether the so-called *hairy ear syndrome* is actually Y-linked or autosomal. The majority support Y-linked, and I agree with them: personally, I've never seen a woman with tufts of hair sprouting out of her ears.

The family tree for a Y-linked condition (*Figure 10*) is, I must confess, a little immodest. In fact, it's mine – because I (indicated by the arrow) am a "victim," if that's the word, of the hairy ear syndrome. As you can see, so were my father, uncle and grandfather. In fact, my father, who knocked around the Middle East a lot, was known there as *Abba Soufle*, which means "Father of the Hairy Ears." You can also see that both my brothers have the condition. I imagine my sons and nephew will, too, when they reach the appropriate age. A family tree containing a Y-linked condition would always look like mine, whether the condition were the hairy ear syndrome or anything else that may prove to be Y-linked. The overriding characteristic, of course, would be that women would never get the condition at all. Not having a Y chromosome, they couldn't. Men would just pass it on to their sons, who would pass it on to their sons, and so on.

Fortunately for me and my sons, the hairy ear syndrome is hardly a threat to one's health. Now we're going to look at some much more serious problems and the families in which they occurred. When we do, I think you'll agree that these families possessed few, if any, things more important than their family trees. But I believe very strongly that the benefits to your family of an accurate, medically detailed family tree could be every bit as great.

Let's now see how some family trees made all the difference to many people's health and happiness today. And to their children's health and happiness tomorrow.

❧ 3 ❧

When The Diagnosis Is in Doubt, Consult Your Family Tree

Perhaps the best way of showing what a great medical asset a family tree can be is to show what can happen without one.

ELLEN: MISERY FROM A MISDIAGNOSIS

Ellen (once again, not her real name) found out about misdiagnosis the hard way. A high-strung girl, she'd always tended to get pretty tense and edgy when the pressure was on. However, she coped fairly well with life, and even picked up a science degree along the way.

Then, in her mid-twenties, she married. For the first year or so, things went well. But after thirteen months of married life, the first baby came along, and all Ellen's latent problems suddenly and traumatically surfaced.

People with no emotional problems often find parenthood a battle. Ellen just couldn't cope with it at all. She tried heroically, but found herself plunging deeper and deeper into depression. Her local doctor, unable to help, arranged for her admission to a psychiatric hospital.

The staff psychiatrists at the hospital tested Ellen, agreed that she was schizophrenic, and gave her shock treatment. It made little or no difference. So Ellen was put on powerful tranquilizers and antidepressant drugs, and released from the hospital.

For some months she battled on – and "battled" was the right word for it. When she first came to me, she was getting nowhere fast. Although still on antidepressants, she was chronically depressed, frequently confused, unable to cope and verging on complete despair.

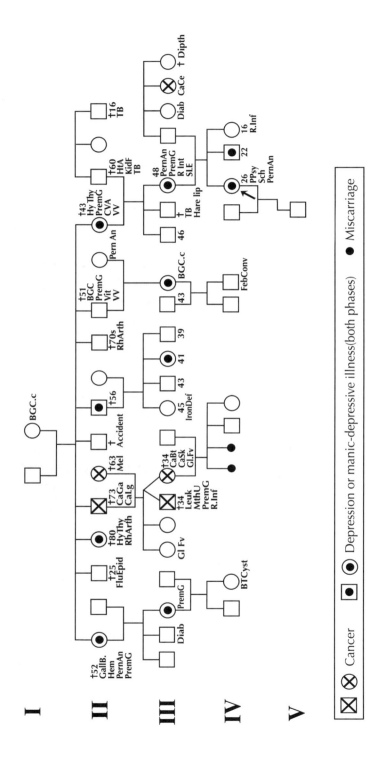

Figure 11: Ellen

A number of very unpleasant problems with a common link: autoimmune disease.

B/G.C.B1	=	Blue/Green color-blind
B/G.C.B1.c	=	Blue/Green color-blind carrier
Bt.Cyst	=	Breast cysts
Ca Bt	=	Breast cancer
Ca Ce	=	Cervical cancer
Ca Ga	=	Gastric (stomach) cancer
Ca Lg	=	Lung cancer
Ca Sk	=	Skin cancer
C V A	=	Cardiovascular accident (stroke)
Diab	=	Diabetes
Dipth	=	Diptheria
Feb Conv	=	Febrile convulsions
Flu Epid	=	Flu epidemic
Gall Bl	=	Gall bladder problems
Gl Fv	=	Glandular fever
Haemd	=	Hemorrhoids
Hare Lip	=	Hare lip & cleft palate

Ht A	=	Heart attack
Hy Thy	=	Hypothyroidism
Iron Def	=	Iron deficiency anemia
Kid F	=	Kidney failure
Leuk	=	Leukemia
Mel	=	Melanoma
Mth U	=	Mouth ulcers
Ov cyst	=	Ovarian cyst
Pern An	=	Pernicious anemia
Prem G	=	Premature graying
P Psy	=	Puerperal psychosis
Rh Arth	=	Rheumatoid arthritis
R Inf	=	Recurrent infections
Sch	=	Schizophrenia
SLE	=	Systemic lupus erythematosus
TB	=	Tuberculosis
Vit	=	Vitiligo
V V	=	Varicose vein

As usual, I started off by getting Ellen to provide a family history. And when she did so, the vital diagnostic clue was clearly revealed.

There were a number of very unpleasant diseases in Ellen's family tree (*Figure 11*), beginning with her mother's pernicious anemia. This is a nasty combination of anemia (bigger-than-usual red blood cells) and a massive Vitamin B_{12} deficiency. If untreated, pernicious anemia can lead to paralysis of the spinal cord, and to premature aging, an early onset of the mental confusion and depression that sometimes accompany old age. Interestingly, its symptoms can be very like those of schizophrenia. There were also indications of pernicious anemia elsewhere in the family. Ellen's great uncle had vitiligo, patches of white skin, which is known to accompany it. Her great aunt, the family recalled, "was required to eat lots of raw liver" – an old treatment for pernicious anemia. The great aunt's son had two other known companions of the disease, diabetes and premature graying. There was more of significance, too. Also in the family tree were rheumatoid arthritis, thyroid trouble, depressive illness, stomach cancer and leukemia.

There's a common link between those illnesses and pernicious anemia. They're all frequently caused by what we call an autoimmune process. In plain English, that means that the body is being distinctly unfriendly to its owner, and is producing antibodies against itself. Those autoimmune antibodies can crop up in almost any part of the body, and cause slow but severe tissue damage wherever they occur. When so many illnesses of that kind occur in a family with pernicious anemia, you can be pretty certain that the family has a genetic tendency to autoimmune disease. So if someone in that family is depressed and confused, you don't just assume they are schizophrenic. You suspect that the family's autoimmune-disease tendency might be rearing its head again. Then you start by testing them for *latent* pernicious anemia, which is the massive Vitamin B_{12} deficiency without the anemia – and which also can produce schizophrenialike symptoms.

So I ran Ellen through the tests. As I expected, she did have latent pernicious anemia. That was the major cause of her psychiatric problem. She didn't have schizophrenia at all. Poor Ellen could have had shock treatment and antidepressants until the cows came home, without ever showing much improvement.

How did the hospital psychiatrists reach such a major misdiagnosis? They didn't think to take a family history. They treated Ellen in isolation, without considering her genetic background. As a result, the relevant tests were simply never done.

Once we knew Ellen's problem, progress was swift. I put her on a course of Vitamin B_{12} injections, with supplements of other vitamins in which she was low. Within eight weeks, her symptoms were vastly improved. She was happily looking after her husband and child. And that wasn't all – shortly afterwards, she became pregnant again. She is now coping splendidly with not one, but two, children. She did suffer a slight relapse some months later when she went off the vitamins, but as soon as she took them again her recovery once more surged ahead.

Her husband told me recently that Ellen is now healthier and happier than she has ever been, for as long as he has known her.

So Ellen's story illustrates a very important principle indeed. By suggesting the most likely diagnosis for your symptoms, your family tree can tell your doctor what tests to do – and greatly lessen the chance of a wrong diagnosis being made.

SUSAN: WHAT DID HER ACHES AND PAINS MEAN?

The point is further underlined by the experience of Susan who was, to put it mildly, not feeling the brightest. The problem that brought her to me was depression, but she did have other symptoms too. Chief among these were a few aches and pains here and there in her body.

The aches and pains, while vague, were persistent. Shortly before she came to me, Susan went to a rheumatologist to have them investigated. The rheumatologist checked Susan over carefully. He discovered osteoarthritis in her knees, but found nothing to explain the vague aches and pains. I wasn't too interested in them at first, because I was concentrating on Susan's depression. But after I saw her family tree (*Figure 12*), the aches and pains suddenly took on a new significance.

Susan's mother, like Susan herself, had arthritis. Susan's maternal uncle and sister both had bowel cancer. That same unfortunate sister also suffered from severe depression, as did the other sister and the maternal aunt.

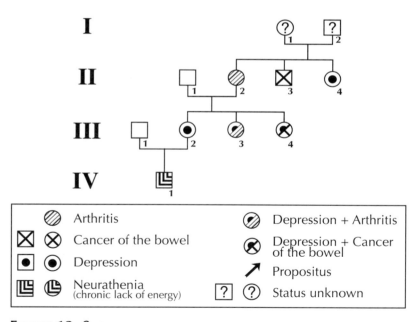

FIGURE 12: Susan

When cancer, arthritis and depression keep bobbing up in a family, you think of SLE.

And Susan's nephew, as you can see, was afflicted with chronic lack of energy. That crop of ailments suggested that here we had another autoimmune-disease family. And it did more. It gave me a very specific diagnostic clue as to the likely basis of Susan's illness.

The family's main problems were cancer, severe depression and arthritis. That particular combination accompanies an unpleasant autoimmune culprit with the jaw-breaking name of systemic lupus erythematosus – usually called just SLE.

SLE is, in fact, a kind of arthritis, although not the normal kind that Susan's rheumatologist was looking for. It is actually a degeneration of the body's connective tissue, the basic tissue that holds you together. It affects the skin and other organs, depending on where it flares up. It produces aches and pains, just like Susan's. And one of its major symptoms is a deep, chronic depression. Just like Susan's. I ran the obvious tests, and obtained the expected results. Susan had SLE. Fortunately, it was in a fairly early stage. I was able to treat it by modifying her diet, rather than by using the cortisone that more advanced cases may demand.

Susan picked up quite quickly. And as her SLE improved, her depression lifted. That wasn't surprising, because the SLE was causing the depression. But if I hadn't seen her family tree, I would never have picked up on the SLE. I would never have linked her aches and pains with her depression – just as the rheumatologist didn't link her aches and pains.

Once again, it was the family tree that suggested the correct diagnosis and indicated the right tests.

BERNARD: PROGRESSIVE BRAIN DAMAGE STOPPED BY A FAMILY TREE

When Bernard came to see me, an accurate diagnosis of his condition was what he needed above everything else. There had been no lack of attempts to provide one. At least eight doctors had sought the reason for his symp-

toms, which had started to appear about three years previously.

The symptoms were severe and alarming. Bernard, a
top executive, could no longer perform any effective
work. He was losing his speech. His balance was very
unsteady. His memory and concentration were leaving
him. He could barely write and he suffered from blinding,
crippling headaches.

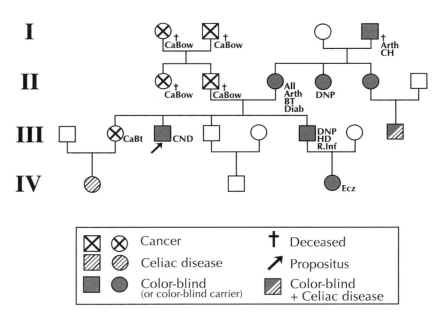

FIGURE 13: BERNARD

Spectacular problems on the X chromosome.

All	= Allergies	C.N.D.	= Central nervous system degeneration
Arth	= Arthritis		
B.T.	= Brain tumor	Diab	= Diabetes
Ca Bow	= Bowel cancer	D.N.P	= Depression, nervous problems
Ca Bt	= Breast cancer		
Ca Ga	= Gastric (stomach) cancer	Ecz	= Eczema
		H.D.	= Headaches
C.H.	= Cerebral hemorrhage	R.Inf	= Recurring infections

After an impressive array of investigations, several diagnoses had been made. They included a brain tumor, meningitis, multiple sclerosis, hydrocephalus (a build-up of fluid on the brain), and encephalitis caused by a reaction to vaccines for an overseas business trip. All were thoroughly tested. All proved negative.

So that was the rather awesome problem that confronted me. And yet, surprisingly, it turned out to be a fairly easy one to solve.

Fortunately, Bernard had a good knowledge of his forebears and was lucid enough to recall them. There was a significant X-linked genetic marker, shining like a beacon, in his mother's family ranks. And a sinister element in his father's family shed extra light on Bernard's situation.

The result is shown in *Figure 13*. The likely cause of Bernard's problem was suddenly clear, although it may take a little explaining.

You can see from the family tree that Bernard himself is red-green color-blind. That's an X-linked recessive condition, and it came to him, as you can also see, through his mother's family. Because his maternal grandfather was color-blind, Bernard's mother and his two aunts had to be carriers (because they received the grandfather's X chromosome, where the condition was located). Bernard's mother passed the offending gene on to him and to Neville, his youngest brother, who is also color-blind. Clive, the middle brother, has perfectly normal vision so he obviously received the mother's other X chromosome, and not the one carrying the color blindness. Clive, in fact, is perfectly healthy. His son is too. Neville, on the other hand, has a depressive anxiety state, bad nerves, headaches and recurring infections. His daughter, who received his color-blind X chromosome and is thus a color-blind carrier, suffers from eczema.

In other words, those who dodge the family's color-blind X chromosome are fit and well. Those who get it tend to have other health problems as well. And that, as you'll note from the family tree, has been happening since granddad's day.

Granddad himself had osteoarthritis and a cerebral hemorrhage. Bernard's mother had arthritis, a brain tumor, diabetes and various allergies. His aunt has nervous problems and depression. His sister, Sarah, has bowel cancer. And so on. What do they all mean? What else on that X chromosome is causing such spectacular problems?

The answer, I felt sure, was being provided by three people – Bernard's cousin, sister and niece. The cousin and niece had both been diagnosed as having celiac disease. That's a condition caused by grain allergies so severe that they actually damage tissues. As soon as I saw it in the family tree, I felt sure it was the X-linked culprit behind most of the family's troubles.

For instance, because it causes tissue damage, it could well have been a factor in Bernard's mother's brain tumor, and his grandfather's cerebral hemorrhage. Because it affects the joints, it could have been behind their arthritis and osteoarthritis. The grain allergies prevent the proper absorption of essential vitamins and minerals, so it could explain brother Neville's and the aunt's depressive problems. It is definitely liked with bowel cancer, such as Bernard's sister Sarah has. It could even be causing his niece's eczema. And because it is known to cause central nervous system degeneration, it most certainly could have been the cause of Bernard's problems.

So, just by looking at Bernard's immediate family and his maternal ancestry, I had my tentative diagnosis; celiac disease. The unpleasant goings-on in the father's family further confirmed it. Bernard's father, aunt and both grandparents on that side had all died of stomach cancer. And as I said before, stomach cancer and celiac disease are known partners in crime. Consequently, there was a strong possibility of celiac disease in the father's family too – and if so, a double inheritance of it for Bernard, Neville, Sarah and the next generation. From every angle, the celiac theory hung together beautifully. The next step was obvious. Test Bernard to see if he did, in fact, have evidence of celiac disease.

I did. And he did. He was massively allergic to grains. As a direct result, he was very low in vitamins and minerals, despite the fact that he took powerful vitamin-mineral supplements regularly. And he had just the kind of autoimmune antibodies that are strong indicators of celiac disease. The diagnostic puzzle was solved – what had eluded medicine's most sophisticated tests yielded immediately to a simple family tree.

Once we knew what was wrong with Bernard, we could do something about it. The treatment consisted of a totally grain-free diet and heavy doses of the vitamins and minerals in which he was so low. In addition, I took him off a tranquilizer-antidepressant that had been part of his medication for months.

These steps may not seem dramatic in the face of such crippling symptoms, but nothing else was required. Within a matter of weeks, Bernard was a whole lot better. There was a noticeable improvement in his speech, writing, balance, coordination and ability to walk. His headaches and stomach upsets were gone. He was sleeping much more soundly. He had considerably more energy, and the white dots in his fingernails (a symptom of Vitamin B_6 and zinc deficiencies) had disappeared.

After five months, I had the pathology tests carried out again. And the results were startling. In that comparatively short time, Bernard's vitamin and mineral deficiencies were eliminated. Even more important, his autoimmune disease had completely cleared up. The autoimmune antibodies were gone.

This meant that his body was free of the components, or fractions, of grain to which he was so allergic, and which, in his case, were so toxic that they were actually causing the damage to his brain and other tissues.

Some damage, of course, had been done before we started. So Bernard may never completely recover his full faculties of speech, balance, coordination and writing. Still, his deterioration had been slowed dramatically. Before he came to me, he was going downhill week by week. The family tree's message halted that. It enabled us to pinpoint the cause of Bernard's brain damage – the grain allergies underlying the celiac disease, and to eliminate it.

So Bernard's family tree has saved him from a future of rapid deterioration and probable early death. And it's opened the door to positive treatment for some of his relatives as well. All because its diagnostic message was so loud and clear.

NANCY: WHEN A FAMILY TREE SPOKE LOUDER THAN TESTS

Sometimes a family tree points to a diagnosis so strongly that you know it has to be right, even when the indicated tests seem, at first, to contradict it. Such was the case with Nancy, who came to me after a succession of doctors had scratched their heads over her failure to respond to treatment.

Nancy had a long history of depression and anxiety, linked with chronic lack of energy, headaches, poor memory and concentration, and arthritis. Virtually all the doctors she had seen – no less than seven in the last few years – had decided that the depression was her basic problem. They had treated her with the appropriate drugs, and experienced the frustration that comes with zero-level results.

One even called in a hypnotherapist, with an equal lack of success. Another sent her to a psychologist, who did at least help her to cope better with the depression.

But the depression itself rumbled on unchecked.

One didn't need to be a stupendous medical genius to realize that all those doctors had been missing something. The question was – what? As soon as I saw Nancy's family tree (*Figure 14*), I was sure I knew the answer.

On Nancy's mother's side, notice the high incidence of cancer, particularly bowel cancer, which had struck Nancy's grandfather, uncle and aunt. Nancy's mother herself suffered from serious bowel disorders, colitis and diverticulitis, and both she and the aunt had severe recurrent depression. The pattern was a classic one for

grain allergies, coming down the generations in an autosomal dominant way.

Then I looked at Nancy's father's family. He suffered
from depression, arthritis and chronic indigestion. His
twin brother had depression and arthritis. Of his other two
brothers, one had arthritis and diverticulitis. Here was
another pattern highly suggestive of grain allergies, this
time with an X-linked dominant transmission. It seemed
certain that hereditary grain allergies had swooped down
on Nancy from both sides of her family. So I immediately
had the appropriate grain allergy tests done.

And they revealed nothing at all.

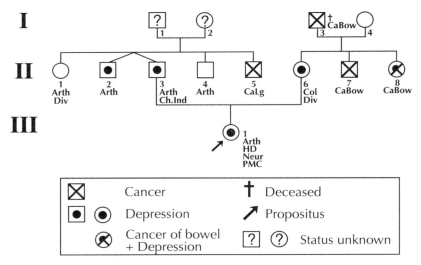

FIGURE 14: Nancy
A classic grain allergy pattern on both sides – despite what the tests
said.

Arth	= Arthritis	H D	= Headaches
Ca Bow	= Bowel cancer	Neur	= Neurasthenia
Ca Lg	= Lung cancer		(chronic lack of
Ch Ind	= Chronic indigestion		energy)
Col	= Colitis	PMC	= Poor memory,
Div	= Diverticulitis		concentration

I remember staring at the results in disbelief. It was like glancing out your window and seeing the sun setting in the east. Then I looked again at the family tree. The patterns were still there. They were still unmistakable. True, no one had ever actually diagnosed grain allergies in Nancy's family, but I still believed that nothing else could produce such a characteristic family tree.

Accordingly, I believed the family tree rather than the tests. I tried again, this time with ingested food allergy tests, covering 84 different foods.

The results? Negative. Not a single allergy showed among the whole lot. I could have stopped at that point and become the eighth baffled doctor in Nancy's recent life.

I didn't stop – the family tree was just too persuasive. But we'd done almost every known food allergy test. Where did we go from there?

Well . . . if it wasn't whole foods, it had to be food components – fractions of grains, perhaps, like gluten and α-gliadin. If they were the culprits, Nancy's system would have produced some very distinctive antibodies in an attempt to combat them. I tried a few other tests, virtually the last shots in our locker, looking for reticulin and bile-duct antibodies.

And this time we hit the jackpot – both tests were most emphatically positive. Just as the family tree had suggested, Nancy was fiercely allergic to grains, or their components, and to milk components as well.

Nancy's problem had finally yielded up its secret, thanks entirely to the persuasive power of her family tree. I put her on a very strict grain- and milk-free diet, and the results confirmed the diagnosis. Nancy started to improve almost immediately. She has made steady progress ever since, as her tissues gradually repair the damage inflicted on them by nonstop allergic reactions.

This underlines another tremendously important benefit flowing from Nancy's family tree. Remember all that bowel cancer running through it? I believe an important cause of that may have been the constant battering of allergic reactions on intestinal tissues. The process was well advanced in Nancy. It has now been halted. She was at very great risk of being her family's next bowel cancer victim. That risk has been cut to a minimum – because of the story told by her family tree.

When Nancy drew up her family tree, she was not only solving her psychiatric problems; in all probability, she was saving her life.

You can't ask much more of a family tree than that.

PAT: WHY SLEEP THERAPY WORKED FOR A WHILE

In the case of Pat, a lady in her early forties, the lack of a family tree had everyone heading up a blind alley for a very long time.

Poor Pat was really in a mess. For 20 years, she had been trapped in a nightmare world of irrationality and confusion. She'd had enough shock treatment and anti-depressants to flatten an elephant. She was averaging nine months a year in the hospital. But she'd never shown more than the slightest improvement.

Eventually, the staff at one hospital decided to try a technique called sleep therapy. As the name implies, this means putting people under heavy sedation, so that they actually sleep for two or three weeks. Throughout the treatment, they are fed intravenously by a glucose drip.

The theory of sleep therapy is that it relieves people of all responsibility for a significant period of time. Everything is done for them. All pressures and stress are removed. It's really a regression to a childhood state of dependence, as well as a complete rest. It gives the sub-conscious mind a chance to sort itself out and resolve the patient's problems. As a result, when the patient wakes up, he or she will be a whole lot better.

That's the theory, anyway. Sometimes it works and sometimes it doesn't. The treatment is not without risk, because of the long duration and depth of sedation. But, in Pat's case, it looked as though it might, indeed, have worked. She really did seem better when she woke up. She was relaxed, rational and happy. The doctors watched with cautious optimism as the first few days passed.

Then, slowly but surely, their optimism turned to puzzled despair. After a few days, Pat's apparent improvement ground to a halt. From that point on, her condition steadily deteriorated. Within a week, she was right back where she had been before the treatment – and where she had been for the last twenty years.

Shortly afterwards, she came into the psychiatric ward of one of Sydney's biggest and most respected hospitals. The medical superintendent concluded that she was a chronic paranoid schizophrenic. Given the facts before him, this was a reasonable diagnosis – even if it did condemn Pat to a bleak and hopeless future.

I saw her soon after that verdict was passed. But what could I do for her, after virtually every weapon of modern psychiatry had failed? Quite a lot, as it turned out, because I could do something that no one else had done in all those twenty years. And that, of course, was to take a family history.

What a revealing family history it turned out to be (*Figure 15*).

It wasn't as detailed as many others I've seen, but there was enough there to show that Pat's twenty years of suffering could have been avoided. Even now, if my intuitions were right, it was going to be fairly easy to help her.

How could I be so sure? The first clue was Pat's mother, who suffered from chronic severe depression, anxiety, irritability and lack of energy. These are typical symptoms of what we learnedly call the *allergic tension fatigue syndrome*, which is caused by food allergies. Pat's mom also had asthma, an allergic complaint, and angina – another condition which many authorities are now linking with food allergies.

Then there was Pat's maternal grandfather. He had suffered from presenile dementia, and had been permanently confined to an institution. As we'll see in Chapter 8, that's commonly caused by pernicious anemia (low Vitamin B_{12}), pellagra (low Vitamin B_3), low Vitamin B_1, low folic acid or an underactive thyroid – all of which are definitely associated with severe food allergies, usually to milk and grains. Finally, to sharpen the picture even further, food allergies had already been diagnosed in two of Pat's cousins.

There are no prizes for guessing what immediately popped into my mind. Food allergies, I was certain, would prove to be the villains behind Pat's ordeal. In many circumstances, they produce psychiatric symptoms that mimic schizophrenia to the last detail.

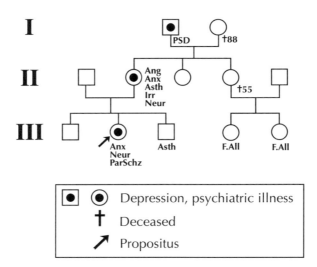

FIGURE 15: **Pat**
The correct diagnosis had eluded everyone for 20 years. The family tree provided it at a glance.

Ang = Angina	Neur = Neurasthenia (chronic lack of energy)
Anx = Anxiety	
Asth = Asthma	Par. Schz = Paranoid schizophrenia
F. All = Food allergies	
Irr = Irritability	PSD = Presenile dementia

So, once again, the family tree suggested a diagnosis which had eluded everyone for twenty years – and showed me what tests to do. Accordingly, I ran a full series of food allergy tests on Pat. The results confirmed what the family tree was saying – and in a quite spectacular way.

Poor Pat had no fewer than eighteen food allergies. Suddenly it was glaringly obvious why the sleep therapy had produced initial results that soon fizzled out. While Pat had been asleep, she hadn't been eating the foods to which she was allergic. So when she woke up, she was free from symptoms. Then, as she resumed eating, all of her old allergic reactions started again and the symptoms returned.

It was a simple as that.

The next step was fairly simple, too – get Pat on a diet that avoided her eighteen food allergies. The results were nothing short of miraculous. Within days, the improvement was obvious. Within weeks, Pat was a normal, rational human being.

She was well again – for the first time in twenty years.

From then on, unfortunately, Pat's story becomes one of ups and downs. She stayed well for about nine months. Then she gradually went off the diet. As she did so, her symptoms began to return. Before long, Pat was entirely off the diet and back in the hospital. At that point, her family managed to get her back onto the diet. She quickly improved. In a short time, she was out of the hospital and feeling fine. Then, a few months later, her strictness with the diet again started to slip.

And that's been the pattern ever since. Whenever Pat relaxes the diet, she becomes psychotic. When she gets back on it, she rapidly improves. But soon she feels so well that the diet seems unnecessary, and the whole cycle starts again.

Despite its roller-coaster history, Pat's case is another vivid illustration of my point: Your family tree can guide your doctor to the right diagnosis – often when all other diagnostic tools have failed – and clearly indicate the tests needed to confirm it.

Consequently, it can save much valuable time and a lot of expensive shooting in the dark. Most importantly, it greatly lessens the chance of a wrong diagnosis being made, and followed up with a useless, and possibly tragic, course of treatment.

If that were the only benefit that a family tree provided, it would still be well worth your while to compile one. Getting a quick, accurate diagnosis of your condition is a flying start toward clearing it up.

But family trees can do a lot more than suggest vital diagnostic clues. In many baffling cases where the right treatment is by no means obvious, even though the diagnosis has been made, the family tree can point the doctor straight toward the correct line of action.

This came home to me forcefully when I began treating the Woodbridge family. They were the ones who started me on the family tree approach, and their remarkable family tree was fascinating in two ways.

First, it suggested a successful line of treatment, which would certainly never have occurred to me otherwise. Second, it vividly illustrates a genetic principle that has, I believe, enormous possibilities for the treatment of, and research into, a whole host of diseases – including such nasties as cancer, schizophrenia, multiple sclerosis and muscular dystrophy. And, surely, anything that might cast new light on that lot is worth looking into.

We'll start doing that now, via the Woodbridge family.

⫷4⫸

How Your Family Tree Can Suggest the Right Treatment

THE WOODBRIDGES: WHERE IT ALL BEGAN

When Joanne Woodbridge walked into my surgery, I certainly had no idea that her case would launch me on a new approach to medicine – and lead eventually to the writing of this book.

Joanne was a middle-aged woman with a long history of manic-depressive illness. That's a condition in which the patient's moods swing wildly between deep depression and a brittle, hyperactive gaiety. Joanne had been in and out of institutions, with more ins than outs, for 35 years.

During that time, they really gave her the works. Insulin coma therapy, shock treatment, antidepressants, lithium, chlorpromazine and haloperidol were just some of the treatments she'd had. But, like so many of the patients I seem to get, Joanne had derived very little benefit from all that nonstop effort.

Early in my first interview with her, I learned that the manic-depressive illness had affected no fewer than five generations of her family, and that "other conditions" were apparently accompanying it. That was interesting, I thought. What could it mean? Might it suggest an answer? How could I investigate it?

Suddenly, I thought of asking Joanne to compile a family tree, and put all the medical information on it that she possibly could. I wasn't sure what it would reveal; but, even then, I felt that some sort of pattern might emerge.

Joanne plunged into the project with gusto. She received valuable help from a number of relatives, especially her 86-year-old mother. This remarkable lady was an active, lucid, highly intelligent ex-lecturer in chemistry, with a Master of Science degree. Most importantly, she had an excellent memory of both her own and her late husband's grandparents and families.

With so much help, a quite outstanding family tree emerged. Although the first, it remains among the best and most detailed I have yet seen (*Figure 16*). And it clearly showed the depressive illness marching through the generations in Joanne's father's family in a frighteningly relentless way.

Joanne's father had suffered from it. So had her paternal grandmother. So had her great-grandfather. Two of her sisters were victims. And, in the next generation, so was her 26-year-old nephew. Five generations in all. But that was only the start.

There were, indeed, other conditions traveling through those five generations. They were red-green color blindness, Xg negative blood group and Vitamin B_{12} deficiency, showing up as pernicious anemia or latent pernicious anemia.

And here was the truly fascinating thing. Every single person in those five generations who suffered from depression also had pernicious anemia or latent pernicious anemia. They were also color-blind and had Xg negative blood (if they were men) or were carriers for those conditions if they were women.

Why was that tremendously significant? Because those three conditions are known to be transmitted genetically in an X-linked way. And here they were, for five generations, appearing in precisely the same people who also had depressive illness.

The conclusion was inescapable. In Joanne's family, the depressive illness was not being caused by environment or stress or upbringing or anything like that. It was being transmitted genetically. What's more, it was on the same X chromosome as the red-green color blindness, the Xg negative blood grouping and the Vitamin B_{12} deficiency.

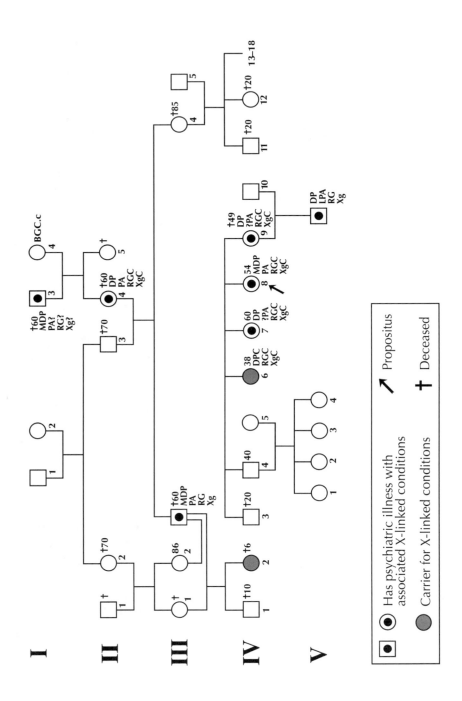

FIGURE 16: the Woodbridge family

The family tree that launched me on the family tree approach to health: five generations of manic-depressive illness, accompanied by three X-linked genetic markers.

Dp	= Depression
DpC	= Carrier for depression, or at risk for it
LPA	= Latent pernicious anemia
PA	= Pernicious anemia
?PA	= Anemia, probably pernicious anemia
PA?	= Pernicious anemia likely, but unknown
MDP	= Manic-depressive illness (bipolar)

RG	= Red-green color-blind male
RG?	= Unknown, but likely to be red/green color-blind male
RGC	= Red/green color-blind female
Xg	= Xg negative blood-group male
Xg?	= Probable Xg negative blood-group male
XgC	= Carrier for Xg negative blood-group

This led immediately to an important train of thought. When we talk about a hereditary Vitamin B_{12} deficiency, what we actually mean is a hereditary metabolic disturbance, which causes the Vitamin B_{12} deficiency. Now, as we have already seen, Vitamin B_{12} deficiencies go hand in hand with depression. But Vitamin B_{12} deficiencies are correctable. So, in Joanne's case, if we corrected the Vitamin B_{12} deficiency, mightn't that also correct the depressive illness?

It was a sound theory. And, better still, it worked in practice.

Joanne has already received years of treatment with lithium carbonate, the standard treatment for manic-depressive illness. I left her on that, and added heavy doses of Vitamin B_{12}. Within weeks, she was out of the hospital for the first time in years.

That was just over four years ago; Joanne has been well ever since – because her family tree pointed us straight toward the correct course of treatment.

What's more, subsequent tests showed that her hereditary metabolic defect was a severe grain allergy. Because of this allergy, her body wasn't able to absorb Vitamin B_{12} properly. Hence the deficiency. So, a strict grain-free diet corrected the deficiency, and enabled the Vitamin B_{12} therapy to be progressively scaled down.

THE X-LINKED PRINCIPLE

Now, here's the point I really want to emphasize. Joanne's depression was curable because it was linked genetically with a curable metabolic defect. When you cured the defect, you cured the illness. And that, I believe, applies not only to X-linked depressive illnesses, but also to a host of others – many cancers, arthritis, diabetes, thyroid disorder, schizophrenia, and pernicious anemia, to name some – and maybe even the risk for multiple sclerosis, as we'll see in Chapter 11.

Typically, you see many families in which a number of these illnesses appear. What is happening then, I believe, is that an X-linked tendency to food allergies, vitamin-mineral deficiencies and autoimmune disease is running through their ranks. It manifests itself in a number of different ways – cancer in some people, arthritis in others, diabetes in still others, and so on.

Consequently, the principle is this: If any of these unpleasant things are running in a family, look for any curable X-linked conditions that might be running with them. Then, treat those conditions, and you'll greatly improve, if not totally cure, the associated illness. I've seen it happen, and I'll have more to say about that in Chapter 11.

The evidence for that genetic link is so strong that all research into cancer, depressive illnesses, psychoses, multiple sclerosis and other serious disorders should be taken into account. I am convinced that the cure rate for many of these illnesses would be much higher if doctors would look for and treat the associated X-linked conditions, such as food allergies, vitamin-mineral deficiencies, and so on.

The way to look for those conditions, of course, is to obtain a detailed family tree.

But what if there are no X-linked conditions? Even then, very often, the family tree can still point directly and unmistakably to the right treatment. Usually it turns out to be a totally unexpected one. And sometimes it dramatically simplifies what looks to be an intractable and tragic case.

CORALIE: PSYCHOSURGERY AVOIDED

That was certainly so with Coralie. The expert opinion in her case dictated a horrifying form of treatment: psychosurgery. Understandably, the prospect terrified her. It was her fear of such a drastic, irreversible step that brought her to seek my opinion.

"Is it true, doctor?" she asked in real anguish. "Do I really have to have it? Can't anything else be done?" Looking at her forbidding list of symptoms, I must confess that, just for a moment, I wondered.

Coralie had been deeply depressed for 10 years, often to the point of suicide. Conventional antidepressants had not only failed to budge her blues, but had given her unpleasant side effects. As well, she ached all over, had poor memory and concentration, lacked energy and came down with infections, mouth ulcers, cold sores, and sinusitis at the drop of a hat. Her sex drive was virtually zero. To top it all, her vision was blurred and she suffered acute discomfort from bright lights and glare. But of all her manifold symptoms, Coralie's bleak, black, suicidal depression was the worst.

Recently, another psychiatrist – the latest of a long line and a professor, no less – had put her on massive doses of a powerful antidepressant called Tolvon (mianserin). She was taking 12 tablets a day, whereas the normal dose is around two or three.

When it became clear that even that huge intake was achieving nothing, the professor told Coralie that psychosurgery was her only hope of relief.

Psychosurgery is every bit as fearful as it sounds. The surgeon actually makes a small lesion in the part of the brain that controls emotion. When it works (it doesn't always) you may, indeed, have your depression relieved, but at the cost of losing a little of your personality. You don't experience depression because you're no longer capable of experiencing it. And some degree of depression, after all, is part of everyone's normal emotional makeup.

Coralie was still trying to come to terms with that numbing advice when she went to a rheumatologist about her aches and pains. He suspected a spinal cord tumor and wanted her to have a myelogram, a procedure in which dye is injected into the space around the spinal cord, and x-rays are taken. With the nightmare of psychosurgery, plus a myelogram, hanging over her head, Coralie could be excused for her feelings of apprehension.

Would she really have to have psychosurgery? I earnestly hoped not, for her sake. So I asked her to get busy on her family tree. And, when I saw it, my hope became a near certainty – because what the family tree was telling us would make psychosurgery and a myelogram about as helpful to Coralie as having her tonsils out.

The story is in *Figure 17*.

As you can see, Coralie's mother had lots of things wrong with her, too, but the significant ones were the arthritis and the psychiatric symptoms – chronic anxiety, with poor memory and lack of concentration. What's more, the same sort of things were affecting the mother's sister. Severe lack of energy, depression, poor memory and concentration and, once again, arthritis. Significant, too, were the manic-depressive psychosis and the cancers in Coralie's other aunts and uncle.

What was the significance of those symptoms? Cast your mind back to the previous chapter, and Susan. There we learned that, when you see a combination of arthritis and psychiatric symptoms in a family, you straightaway think of SLE – that particularly nasty form of connective tissue degeneration. SLE also produces a deep, lasting depression and, in addition, overall aches and pains, another of Coralie's major symptoms.

So, once again, a five-minute glance at the family tree suggested a tentative diagnosis, one that hadn't crossed anybody's mind over Coralie's 10-year ordeal. And why hadn't it? Because no one had thought of looking at her family tree.

They had all said, in effect, "Right – this woman is depressed. Let's treat the depression." Incredibly, no one had asked, "Why is she so depressed? What's causing it? How can we discover the cause? And how can we treat it?" When you're ready to ask those questions, the family tree is where you start looking for answers.

Meanwhile, back with Coralie, tests quickly revealed what I knew they would – that she indeed had SLE. What was more, it was severe. She was literally full of autoimmune antibodies. She had antibodies to her connective tissue, her white blood cells and lots of other things. The damage even showed up in a skin biopsy. So now we knew for sure what was causing her depression and aches and pains and all the rest.

The next question was obvious. How could we treat it?

Certainly not by psychosurgery, that was for sure. You don't cure SLE by carving up people's brains.

My first task, and a happy one, was to assure Coralie that psychosurgery was totally unnecessary. And, as the reason for her aches and pains was now abundantly clear, so was a myelogram.

My second task was to ponder over something else that showed up in the tests. As well as her autoimmune antibodies, Coralie had some very bad allergies, particularly to components of milk and grains. The allergies lent extra weight to a theory that was growing in my mind – that SLE might frequently have an allergic base. Here was

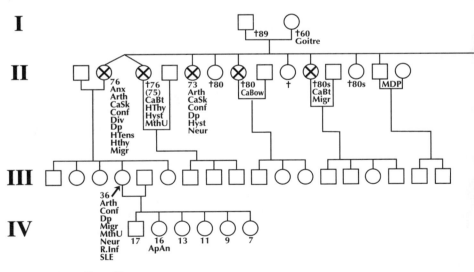

FIGURE 17: Coralie

Psychosurgery avoided – thanks to the clues provided by this family tree.

Anx	= Anxiety	Ca Bt	= Breast cancer
Ap An	= Aplastic anemia as child	Ca Sk	= Skin cancer
Arth	= Arthritis	Conf	= Confusion
Ca Bow	= Bowel cancer	Div	= Diverticulitis

yet another instance of the two things bobbing up together. I was sure it wasn't coincidence.

On the basis of the tests suggested by the family tree, I not only had a definite diagnosis, but a line of treatment, too. That very day, I took Coralie off every food containing milk or grains. That's more easily said than done, but Coralie was sufficiently motivated by the fear of psychosurgery to stick to a very strict diet.

Secondly, I noted that her tests also showed marked vitamin and mineral deficiencies, even though she was regularly taking Vitamin B and C supplements and some minerals. This wasn't really surprising. The allergies were preventing Coralie from properly absorbing vitamins and minerals from her food, and the supplements weren't enough to make up the deficit. So, step two was

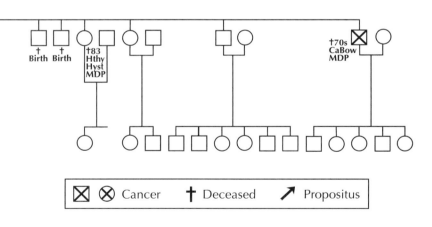

Dp	= Depression	M D P	= Manic-depressive illness
H Tens	= Hypertension	Neur	= Neurasthenia
H Thy	= Hypothyroidism		(chronic lack of energy)
Hyst	= Hysterectomy	R.Inf	= Recurring infections
Migr	= Migraine	S L E	= Systemic lupus erythemotosus
Mth U	= Mouth ulcers		

to put her onto vitamin and mineral supplements strong enough to bridge the gap.

Step number three expressed my confidence that we were on the right track. I immediately scaled down her whopping doses of antidepressants, with firm instructions to cut them out completely in a matter of days. Then we sat back and waited for results.

They weren't long in coming. In just a couple of weeks, Coralie was definitely starting to get better. And from that point on, her improvement simply bounded ahead. Her depression melted away like morning mist. Her aches and pains disappeared. Her eye problems cleared up. She had lots more energy. Her memory and concentration improved. And her rate of picking up infections fell to around the normal level.

It was, quite simply, a staggering improvement. Nor was it a flash in the pan. Coralie has now been well, at the time of this writing, for over three years. All her symptoms, including the deep depression, have been controlled by nothing more than a diet that avoided her allergies, plus relevant vitamins and minerals.

No psychiatric medication, no antidepressants of any kind were necessary. And she needed psychosurgery, literally, like she needed a hole in the head.

Twelve months later, I had all her pathology tests redone. The results were as dramatic as her improvement. Her vitamin and mineral readings were now normal. Even more significant, her extremely high levels of autoimmune antibodies – in her case, the kind that point to SLE – had completely disappeared. Coralie no longer had SLE. Not a trace of it.

Since it was the SLE that had caused all her problems, it was hardly surprising that she was now quite better. Obviously, her SLE had indeed been caused by her massive milk-and-grain-components allergies. By protecting her from them and repairing their effects, we had overcome the SLE. And by overcoming the SLE, we had overcome her psychiatric and physical symptoms.

It sounds easy – but no one had hit on it for 10 long, agonizing years.

A HAPPY BONUS

Meanwhile, there was the problem of Coralie's mother and aunt. Their symptoms, you will recall, were quite like Coralie's, although neither was as bad as she was. It was a safe bet that the family's allergic tendencies were at work in them, too, and so it proved to be. When I tested them, they both had the same milk-grain-component allergies as Coralie had. They didn't have SLE, but the effects of the allergies were certainly knocking them around.

I sent them off in Coralie's footsteps – onto the same grain- and milk-free diet, plus the relevant vitamins and minerals, that had transformed her life. And it happened again. Within a few months, both ladies' psychiatric and physical symptoms had cleared up.

That was certainly a happy bonus. The family tree's clear message had brought healing to other family members, apart from the original patient: A gratifying result that frequently accompanies the family-tree approach.

Sadly, the insight had come too late for those who had cancer, because I believe that cancer is very often another manifestation of the same food allergy/vitamin-mineral deficiency/autoimmune disease syndrome. We'll look at that theory in detail in Chapters 7 and 11.

It's great that Coralie is well now. Yet, I find her case a disturbing one.

Why? Because it's chilling to think that, but for her family tree, Coralie would have had psychosurgery. A little bit of her personality would have been cut away. And, because psychosurgery doesn't cure SLE, she would have been no better at all.

How many times has that happened in the past? How many times will it happen again – because doctors don't think to take family histories, and read the clear messages they contain?

I repeat – so often, those messages do indicate the right line of treatment for an apparently baffling case. Few people would agree more emphatically with that than Zelda, whose story is a particularly fascinating example of what I'm talking about.

ZELDA: HOW A FAMILY TREE SAVED AN UNBORN BABY

Zelda's family tree certainly suggested a radically new, and dramatically successful, treatment for her. As usual, the treatment would never have entered anyone's head without the family tree's guidance. And it had a very happy side effect: It saved the life of her unborn baby.

When she came to me, Zelda was two months pregnant. But that was hardly a cause for rejoicing. In fact, she had just been told that she would have to terminate the pregnancy. Right away. The bearer of that happy news was a renal, or kidney-function, specialist. He was quite justified in his advice, as Zelda was suffering from chronic kidney failure. It was very doubtful whether her kidneys would stand up to a pregnancy. The termination was necessary, the specialist believed, to save Zelda's life. He had also advised her to have an immediate kidney biopsy, to confirm the diagnosis of renal failure, and prescribed solid doses of cortisone to postpone the inevitable need for a kidney transplant.

But massive though it was, the renal problem was only one of Zelda's ailments. She was also deeply depressed, very pale and anemic, chronically tired, fearful, confused and unable to concentrate. Her sex drive and general motivation for living had all but dried up. And, if asked to make a decision, she felt like diving under the bed.

Not a happy combination of symptoms for Zelda or her husband and two young daughters. What was behind it all? Just the kidney failure? The kidney failure plus depression? Or something more basic still?

Whatever it was, the kidney failure overshadowed everything else. Once the kidneys start to pack it in like that, there's not a lot you can do. True, you can retard the process with cortisone. And kidney transplants are working better all the time. But the prospects ahead of Zelda still weren't very promising.

Those ahead of her unborn baby were even less hopeful.

Anyway, I asked Zelda to compile a family tree. I wasn't, I must admit, too confident that solutions would emerge. She was a very sick woman, and I had a horrible feeling that it might have been too late – if not for her, certainly for the unborn baby.

The family tree arrived. I looked at it, and suddenly I felt like a shipwrecked sailor who sees a rescue ship come steaming over the next wave.

Look at Zelda's family tree (*Figure 18*), and you'll see what I saw. Known food allergies, and conditions suggesting them, running through both sides of her family in a virtually unbroken stream. See them? Both her parents, then Zelda herself, her sister and two brothers. And, as I was later to discover, Zelda's two daughters as well.

Now that's a fairly frightening family tree. I knew, without testing, that Zelda was also going to be awfully allergic. There were only three questions: To what, exactly, was she allergic? What bearing did the allergies have on her legion of problems? And, in particular, did they say anything at all about the kidney failure?

At first sight, the answer to the last question seemed to be "no." The food allergies had battered the last two generations without causing any kidney trouble. But, then I saw two other things that really made me stop and think.

First, Zelda's elder brother also had failing kidneys. Indeed, he was already on permanent cortisone. And second, the food allergies were running on each side of Zelda's family, which meant that she and her brothers and sister may well have copped food-allergy genes from both their mother and their father. If so, and if their allergies turned out to be what I suspected they were, that unhappy doubling up would explain why kidney failure

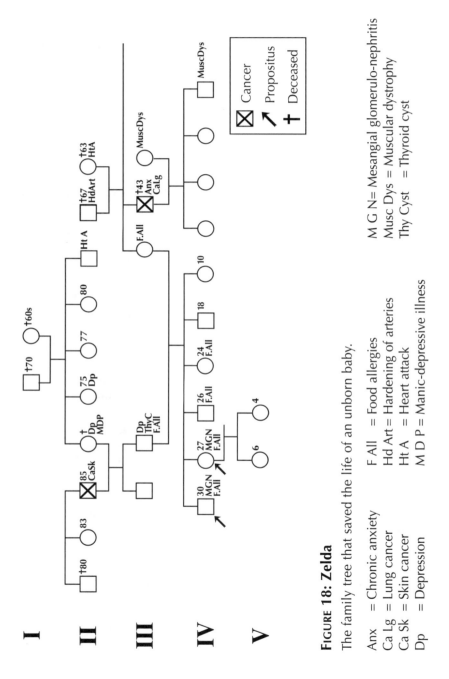

FIGURE 18: Zelda

The family tree that saved the life of an unborn baby.

Anx   = Chronic anxiety
Ca Lg = Lung cancer
Ca Sk = Skin cancer
Dp   = Depression

F All = Food allergies
Hd Art = Hardening of arteries
Ht A   = Heart attack
M D P = Manic-depressive illness

M G N= Mesangial glomerulo-nephritis
Musc Dys = Muscular dystrophy
Thy Cyst = Thyroid cyst

had bobbed up in this generation, and not in previous ones. With all that in mind, I ran the tests to find out just what Zelda's food allergies were.

They turned out to be severe grain allergies. My suspicions were confirmed. Left untreated, grain allergies will, over the years, damage tissues progressively in key areas of the body – including, in some people, the kidneys, where they can even cause such conditions as glomerulonephritis. They will also prevent the patient from properly absorbing vitamins, particularly the B group. The result is a massive and chronic vitamin B deficiency.

And the main symptoms of that? Depression, confusion, tiredness, lack of motivation – everything that was making Zelda's life a misery. It was clear that we had found the problem behind the ailments. The grain allergies were causing both Zelda's kidney failure and her psychiatric symptoms.

That immediately suggested a course of action. Get Zelda totally off the grains to which she was so allergic. Then, back that up with heavy supplements of the vitamins that she was failing to absorb.

Such a line of treatment would certainly overcome the depression. But what about the kidneys? Conventional medical wisdom has it that, once the kidneys are going, that's it. Anything you do only postpones the inevitable.

So you won't find the medical books telling you to treat kidney failure with diet and vitamins. Yet that's exactly what I proposed to do. And I was confident that it would work.

In fact, I was so confident that I advised Zelda not to have her pregnancy terminated. She agreed. I put her on a strict grain-free diet and started the vitamin supplements. Then there was nothing left to do except wait.

While we waited, I pondered further on the family situation. Zelda and her elder brother both had kidney problems . . . both were allergic to grains. What were the implications for the next brother and sister, who were younger but also very allergic to grains? Quite obviously, they were highly at risk for kidney failure in a few years' time, if their grain intake stayed at a high level.

Further down the time trail, a similar peril awaited Zelda's two daughters. Both had inherited grain allergies in full measure. As a result, the six-year-old already had a lot of gastric upsets, headaches and recurring infections. The four-year-old had a milk allergy as well, and suffered from eczema.

This embattled family certainly provided plenty of material for pondering. The question was: Could I, by following the family tree's lead, do anything more concrete for them than that?

As the weeks went by, the happy answer became more and more evident. Zelda's improvement was rapid and obvious in the psychiatric area. Her depression lightened, her confusion melted away, her tiredness and anxiety receded. And, even more important, when the time came for her next kidney tests, the news could hardly have been better. Zelda's kidney functions were actually stabilizing. In fact, many of the test results were completely normal. The anemia had lifted. There would be no need for kidney biopsies or cortisone.

The conclusion was clear. In Zelda and her family, the kidney failure was simply a manifestation of the family's unusually severe grain intolerance. The evidence for that was right before our eyes. Zelda was now totally off grains, and her kidneys were improving – which kidneys usually don't do when they are damaged by disease, degeneration or drugs.

The family tree approach had done it again. It had revealed the basic cause of a very sick lady's complex problems. Then, it had indicated a new line of treatment. And the treatment had worked. That, of course, was great news for Zelda. It was great news, too, for the members of her family. Her brother's kidney failure could now be treated, and he was later able to come off cortisone. Her other brother, her sister and her children now had every chance of avoiding kidney problems before they started.

Zelda's youngest brother and sister, who weren't yet showing grain allergies, received a clear message to cut down on grains before the allergies could develop.

And, because Zelda was recovering, her unborn baby would have a chance to live.

The months passed. After an uneventful pregnancy, Zelda gave birth to a bouncing baby girl. She was even able to breastfeed her. And the fascinating thing was this: despite the baby's allergy-ridden family background, she was completely healthy and infection-free – and remains so, three years later.

Getting Zelda off the grains at an early stage of the pregnancy had obviously been extremely beneficial for the baby's development. It's a little early to say yet, but I think she has an excellent chance of escaping the grain allergies altogether.

So the treatment suggested by Zelda's family tree not only worked, it sent its healing touch through two generations. Zelda, in fact, now has a healthy little boy as well as the three daughters, and all are getting on splendidly.

HEATHER: A BREAKTHROUGH IN A BAFFLING ILLNESS

Kidney problems like Zelda's are very nasty. But at least they're relatively common and well understood. When Heather came to see me, she not only had a cluster of nasty problems, but a condition that was both extremely rare and very mysterious.

It's called primary biliary cirrhosis, and I'll bet you haven't heard of that one. Doctors have, of course, but we'd much prefer *not* to hear about it. What happens in primary biliary cirrhosis is that the liver tissue is gradually replaced by useless fibrous tissue. No one knows what causes it. Worse still, no one is too sure how to treat it.

Or, rather, no one was too sure, until Heather produced a family tree (*Figure 19*) that just might be pointing us toward some answers.

The first thing to emerge from it was that the primary biliary cirrhosis wasn't hers alone. Her brother had a similar condition in the bile ducts. What's more, her son had fibrosis of the lungs. In each case, normal healthy tissue was just changing into nonfunctional fibrous tissue. And as I said, that is extremely rare.

To have it occur three times in two generations in the one family is even rarer. The only possible explanation, apart from wild coincidence, is some sort of genetic factor slinking through the family. Now, for all its slinkiness, such a factor usually betrays itself with some kind of genetic marker. Sure enough, a closer scan of Heather's family tree revealed a telltale pattern.

Take a look for yourself. Here was another terribly allergic family. Food allergies were charging down the generations on both sides – and, as happened with Zelda's family, the two allergic heredities combined in Heather's generation, to make her, her brother and her son the worst-hit of all.

Having noted all that, I formed a theory.

Here was a family with three cases, in two generations, of a very rare illness – plus an extremely high rate of food allergies. Wasn't it at least possible that those two unusual characteristics were linked, that the allergies were, in fact, causing the tissue changes? It seemed a pretty good theory to me. The next step was to test it. I launched into a detailed series of tests to identify Heather's allergies precisely. Heather proved to be very allergic to grains, eggs and milk. As a result, she was extremely deficient in Vitamin B_6, niacin and vital minerals like calcium – which explained her depression. She also had alarmingly high levels of what are known as IgM, mitrochondrial and reticulin antibodies. Her body had produced these in response to the allergies, and their high level was another pointer to the allergies' severity.

It was those allergies, according to my theory, that were damaging Heather's body and causing the primary biliary cirrhosis. Now that they had been identified, the

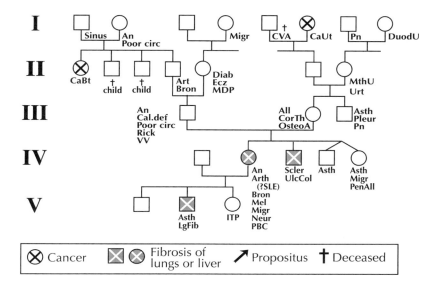

Figure 19: Heather

An extremely rare condition occurring three times in two
generations – coincidence, or genetics?

All	= Allergies	Mth U	= Mouth ulcers
An	= Anemia	Neur	= Neurasthenia
Art	= Arteriosclerosis		(chronic lack of
Arth	= Arthritis		energy)
Bron	= Bronchitis	P B C	= Primary biliary
Ca Bt	= Breast cancer		cirrhosis
Ca Ut	= Uterine cancer	Osteo A	= Osteoarthritis
Cal Def	= Calcium deficiency	Pen All	= Penicillin allergy
Cor Th	= Coronary	Pleur	= Pleurisy
	thrombosis	Pn	= Pneumonia
CVA	= Cardiovascular	Poor circ	= Poor circulation
	accident (stroke)	Rick	= Rickets
Diab	= Diabetes	Scler Chol	= Sclerosing
Duod U	= Duodenal ulcer		cholangitis
Ecz	= Eczema		(fibrosing of bile
ITP	= Low blood platelet		ducts)
	count	Sinus	= Sinusitis
Lg Fib	= Lung fibrosis	SLE	= Systemic lupus
M D P	= Manic-depressive		erythematosus
	illness	Ulc Col	= Ulcerative colitis
Mel	= Melanoma	Urt	= Urticaria (hives)
Migr	= Migraine	VV	= Varicose veins

real test of my theory could be made. I immediately put Heather on a strict diet that avoided grains, eggs, milk and other foods to which she was allergic, like peanuts, black pepper and gelatin. As well, I prescribed solid doses of Vitamin B_6, Vitamin B_{12}, niacin, calcium and other vitamins and minerals that were being drained from her by the allergies.

After just a few weeks, the response was quite dramatic. There was a marked improvement in Heather's liver function. The tissue degeneration had clearly been halted. Moreover, her depression, lack of energy and headaches were much better as well.

Subsequent tests have confirmed the liver improvement. In fact, there are grounds for believing that the tissue degeneration is actually being reversed. If so, this will be, to my knowledge, one of the first cases of primary biliary cirrhosis in the world to be successfully treated without hospitalization or drugs.

Now, that is nothing less than a breakthrough. And, of course, it has exciting implications for Heather's brother and son. Almost certainly, in light of the family history, their fibrous tissue problems are being caused by the same group of food allergies. So now we know what to do to help them as well. And not only them, but also many others in the same situation, because I believe that Heather's family tree shows us a whole new way of looking at a very baffling illness.

I'm not rushing in to claim that every case of primary biliary cirrhosis and its relatives is allergy-based, but shouldn't the possibility always be considered? Shouldn't it now be standard procedure, at least, to take a family history to see if allergies are working their silent sabotage in past and present generations?

For that matter, if clues to an ailment as mysterious as primary biliary cirrhosis can come from a family history, isn't the family tree approach worth trying in every difficult case? Shouldn't doctors, as a matter of course, check to see if allergies, vitamin-mineral deficiencies or other treatable genetically linked metabolic disorders are running in the patient's family?

They should. But at the moment, generally speaking, they aren't.

So, for the time being at least, it's up to you as the patient. If you, or someone in your family, have a problem that is puzzling the doctors, take the initiative. Draw up a good family tree (Chapter 6 shows you how). Look for the patterns and conditions that are genetic clues to the problem (Chapters 7 and 10 will help you there). Point them out to your doctor.

A new – and, possibly, quite unexpected – line of treatment for you could very well emerge.

5

Foretell the Future with Your Family Tree

There's still another way in which a family tree can help your doctor. And this, I often think, is the most exciting way of all.

Your family tree is a kind of time machine. It lets you peer into the future. It shows you, quite clearly, the people in your family who are at risk for certain illnesses. And it sounds the warnings years in advance: plenty of time for something to be done by way of prevention or cure.

Let me illustrate the point, once again from the invaluable Woodbridge family tree.

The Woodbridges, you'll recall, started our previous chapter. Joanne Woodbridge was the fourth of five generations of her family to suffer from depressive illness – which was linked in each generation with red-green color blindness, Xg negative blood group and pernicious anemia.

The fifth generation depressive sufferer was Joanne's nephew Roger. As well as being depressed, he was red-green color-blind. Both conditions had previously occurred in his maternal grandfather (Joanne's father), so Roger had obviously inherited them on an X chromosome. But the grandfather had also had pernicious anemia, and this, as we have seen, was running through the family on the same X chromosome. Roger, in consequence, was clearly very much at risk for pernicious anemia. I had the tests done. Sure enough, Roger had the marked Vitamin B_{12} deficiency that means latent pernicious anemia. However, it could be treated quite easily at this early stage with Vitamin B_{12} injections. As a result, Roger will now avoid true pernicious anemia, with all its shattering effects – and as a bonus, because of the genetic link between the two, his depression should be greatly helped as well.

There was another question, of course: What was causing Roger's Vitamin B_{12} deficiency? The most likely answer, in light of his Aunt Joanne's history, was grain allergies, which prevent the body from absorbing Vitamin B_{12} in the normal way. Further tests revealed that Roger was indeed very allergic to grains. On a strict grain-free diet, he will only need the B_{12} injections temporarily, instead of once a month for the rest of his life.

VALERIE: NO ONE GUESSED WHAT AWAITED HER CHILDREN

Valerie's experience provides another good example of a family tree foretelling the future.

"It's all in your mind," she'd been told by an endocrinologist. Valerie had gone to him for an adrenal function test, prompted by her chronic lack of energy, frequent infections, general aches and pains, recurring diarrhea and depression. Finding nothing, he concluded that her problems were psychological – probably brought on by the stress of caring for three very active children.

I knew her problems certainly weren't "all in her mind." In fact, they turned out to be very physical indeed. Valerie had SLE, and the clue to picking it up was a family tree (*Figure 20*) full of pointers on both sides to food allergies and autoimmune disease.

But even as I set about devising treatment for Valerie, something was nagging at my mind. Those three very active children – what was the family tree telling me about them? Was it performing its time-machine role, and sending out warnings about their future?

To find out, I suggested that the children be tested for food allergies, the prime culprit lurking in the family tree. Valerie agreed. The tests were done and the warnings were there, stark and clear. It was like looking through a window on tomorrow.

All three children had the same group of food allergies as Valerie had. And her food allergies were very closely linked with her SLE. She had, in fact, developed SLE because her food allergies had prevented her body from absorbing certain vitamins and minerals, especially those necessary for a normal immune system. Furthermore, part of her immune system had been directly suppressed by the allergies. Those two effects had led to the development of autoantibodies – antibodies hostile to her own body tissues – which, in conjunction with the food allergies, were causing the SLE. So, if her children had the same food allergies, they were obviously in great danger of developing SLE as well.

Further tests were clearly called for. I carried them out, and found that Valerie's children were already showing signs of various immune system defects, including autoantibodies to various tissues and organs – the early warning indicators of SLE.

However, the warnings came in time.

I put the children on a strict diet, to avoid the foods or, more accurately, the food components, to which they were allergic. The guilty food components in this case appeared to be albumin and globulin fractions (especially of cow's milk, eggs, beef and grains) and gluten and *α-gliadin* grain fractions. As a result, the children's bodies will now properly absorb vitamins and minerals. Their stomach cells, pancreatic ducts and bile ducts, which were starting to reel under the food allergies' assaults, will recover. Their production of traitorous autoantibodies will cease, and they're most *unlikely* to develop SLE.

That happy result is entirely due to their family tree. Without its ability to foretell the future, neither I nor anyone else would have suspected their potential for developing SLE – until the disease was well and truly established.

There's a bonus with their treatment, too, just as there was with Roger's. They were regarded, you will remember,

as being "very active" children. In fact, they were hyperactive, and avoiding their food allergies will control that
condition as well.

I just can't overemphasize the importance of this *time-
machine* effect. In the last few years, I've seen it point a

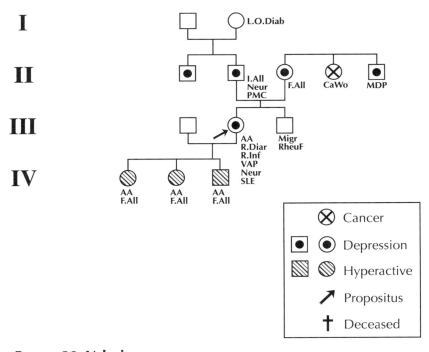

FIGURE 20: Valerie

A *time-machine* family tree that warned of problems ahead for her
three children.

AA	= Autoimmune antibodies	P M C	= Poor memory and concentration
Ca Wo	= Cancer of womb		
F All	= Food allergies	R Diar	= Recurring diarrhea
I All	= Inhalant allergies	Rheu F	= Rheumatic fever
LO Diab	= Late-onset diabetes	R Inf	= Recurring infections
M D P	= Manic-depressive	SLE	= Systemic lupus erythematosus
Migr	= Migraine		
Neur	= Neurasthenia (chronic lack of energy	V A P	= Vague aches, pains illnes

warning finger at apparently normal children so often that I really want to drive the point home. If there are problems running in your family, and their mode of transmission indicates that your children are next in line, for goodness' sake have them tested. It's so easy – and the benefits for their future are incalculable.

JACK: THREE HEALTHY CHILDREN – OR WERE THEY?

Jack's children provide another classic example. He was the chap we met in our introduction – the country professional man who actually had allergic encephalitis, but whose symptoms had everyone chasing after nonexistent brain tumors and nervous breakdowns.

His family tree, you'll remember, cut through the confusion and pinpointed the problem. And a fascinating family tree it is, too. Let's take a look at it in *Figure 21*.

Jack's mother, as you can see, has severe allergies to grains, especially rye, and milk. His maternal grandmother died of Hodgkin's disease and his uncle died of leukemia, two forms of cancer. His maternal great aunt and great uncle both died of pernicious anemia. And it is known that there is a higher rate of cancer and pernicious anemia in families with severe grain allergies and celiac disease. It was very likely, therefore, that milk and grain allergies had plagued the family for generations, which immediately brought them under suspicion of being the culprits in Jack's case. And so it turned out to be.

Jack's main problem was a giant allergy to grains, including wheat and wheat dust; and there he was, living in the heart of an Australian wheat-growing district, where wheat dust wafted around on every breeze. As you'll recall, we put him on a grain- and milk-free diet and filled him with relevant vitamins and minerals, to help repair the damage caused by the allergic reactions. Jack picked up in no time and made a full recovery.

Now that was a good result. But I wasn't happy to leave it there. Jack had three children, all seemingly in good health. However, if the family's allergic tendencies were being passed on in an autosomal dominant fashion, as they appeared to be, all three children faced severe health risks in the future.

That was the clear warning being issued by the family tree's time-machine function. Why not check it out now, while the sun was shining – and before any major health problems surfaced? I put the question to Jack and his wife. They agreed. It proved to be one of the best decisions regarding their children's welfare they'd ever made.

The eldest child, 11-year-old Vanessa, turned out to have a formidable list of grain allergies – among the most daunting that I've yet seen. She was acutely allergic to wheat, yeast, corn, malt, barley, oats and rye. She was also allergic to milk, peanuts, chicken, eggs and cashews. Just to complete the picture, she had a few inhalant allergies to things like molds, grasses and cat fur as well. Vanessa was apparently in good physical health. She was, however, a very sensitive and emotional girl who was easily upset. Now we knew why, and we had a sharply focused picture of her likely future. Vanessa's list of allergies pointed strongly to one diagnosis: celiac disease. As we learned in the last chapter, celiac disease can cause tissue damage. It can also produce psychiatric symptoms in a high percentage of sufferers.

Considering her tantrums and touchiness now, Vanessa faced a real risk, I believe, of a psychotic breakdown in her teens. Added to that was a considerably higher than usual chance of getting arthritis, cancer of the bowel or breast and pernicious anemia in later life – all of which occur much more frequently in people with severe grain allergies.

Advance warning of that little lot are, I think you'll agree, well worth having. The family tree gave them to us. Now, a strict regime of diet, plus relevant vitamins and minerals (to help patch up the damage already done), should make Vanessa no more vulnerable than anyone else to any of those nasties.

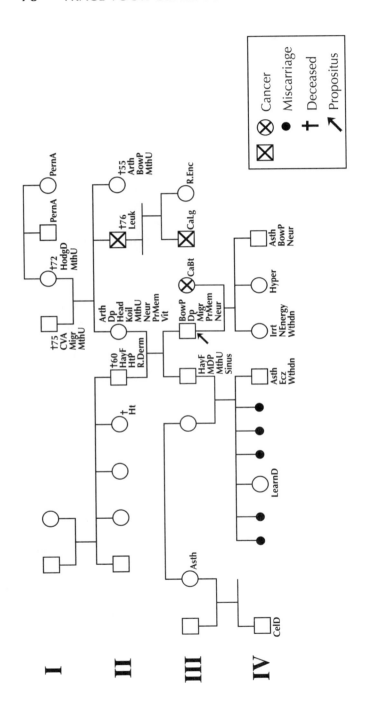

Figure 21: Jack's family

Generations of serious illnesses, linked to milk and grain allergies – with the present generation right in the firing line.

Arth	= Arthritis	Ht P	= Heart problems
Asth	= Asthma	Hodg D	= Hodgkin's disease
Bow P	= Bowel problems	Hyper	= Hyperactivity
Ca Bt	= Breast cancer	Irrit	= Irritable
Ca Lg	= Lung cancer	Koil	= Koilonychia
Cel D	= Celiac disease	Learn D	= Learning difficulties
C V A	= Cardiovascular accident (stroke)	Leuk	= Leukemia
		M D P	= Manic-depressive illness
Dp	= Depression	Migr	= Migraine
Ecz	= Infantile eczema	Mth U	= Mouth ulcers
Hay F	= Hayfever	Neur	= Neurasthenia (chronic lack of energy)
Head	= Headache		

N energy	= No energy
Pern An	= Pernicious anemia
Pr Mem	= Poor memory
R Derm	= Recurrent dermatitis
R Enc	= Recurrent encephalitis
Sinus	= Sinusitis
Vit	= Vitiligo
Wthdn	= Withdrawn

A similar, if less spectacular, story emerged with the two other children – Tracey, aged nine, and Paul, aged seven. Tracey, described by her parents as a "restless" sort of girl, had quite a severe milk allergy, plus inhalant allergies to molds. Left untreated, she had a high risk of developing ulcerative colitis, eczema and asthma, all of which can result from milk allergies.

Paul came somewhere in between Vanessa and Tracey in the seriousness of his condition. Like Vanessa, he had milk and wheat allergies, although they weren't quite as bad as hers. The disturbing thing, however, was that he already suffered from bowel frequency. This indicated that the allergic reactions were irritating his intestinal tissues, the first step in a long process that very often leads to celiac disease and cancer of the bowel. Fortunately, that process can be reversed if Paul avoids milk and wheat like the plague. And under his parents' supervision, he's doing just that. So, once again, his risk of getting celiac disease and bowel cancer should shrink to entirely normal levels.

One very interesting point in this family is that Vera, Jack's wife, has already had a breast removed because of cancer. And as we've just seen, breast cancer has a known association with grain allergies. Consequently, it could well be that grain allergies are running in Vera's family, too, which could mean that Vanessa, Tracey and Paul have received a double dose of dominant allergy genes. That would certainly explain the massive nature of Vanessa's allergies, and why all three are so allergic.

Be that as it may, the point is that no one would normally have suspected the potential for problems lurking within those children. But thanks to the family tree and its time-machine function, the lurkers were unmasked. And we had plenty of time to take corrective action. That's a million times better than trying to cure the illness after it's erupted.

THE RANSOMES: TRAGEDY, THEN HEALING

The family tree's time-machine effect also threw a healing light on the Ransome family's problems – but not before a senseless, totally preventable tragedy had marred their lives.

Iris Ransome had battled against depression for as long as she could remember. A strong-willed, highly intelligent person, she has learned to cope with it. She had reached middle age, having married and raised three children, Geoff, Trevor and Shirley along the way.

The children were now grown up. Unfortunately, Trevor and Shirley both had their mother's depressive illness problem. Both had seen psychiatrists, who had labeled them as *schizophrenics* (when in doubt, call the patient "schizophrenic." It's the handiest label psychiatry has).

Then, purely by accident, Iris stumbled onto exactly the right treatment for her children. She read an article on vitamin therapy, written by a very eminent Australian doctor, and she started giving Trevor and Shirley large doses of various vitamins, particularly Vitamin C.

They both improved quite markedly. Shirley even married and had a son, Trent. But she still wasn't completely well. So in 1973, Iris took Shirley to another psychiatrist.

This person, who certainly has a lot to answer for, was told about the vitamin approach. And he didn't approve. In fact, he ridiculed it. Iris felt so humiliated that she advised Shirley to give up the vitamins. Shirley did so. Her condition rapidly deteriorated. Soon after, she committed suicide.

It was several years later that Iris came to me. She recounted the sad story of Shirley's suicide. I shared her anger and bitterness toward the ignorant, prejudiced doctor who had so tragically misled her. But that was in the past. We had to look at the future – focused in the persons of Trevor and Trent.

Now nine years old, Trent rarely knew what it was to feel well. He was a chronically tired, pale little boy who came down with ear and respiratory infections, hives, abdominal pains and bowel disorders on a depressingly regular basis.

One way or another, the whole Ransome family wasn't exactly living on Cloud Nine. It was clear that some genetic misfortune was running through their ranks, and I already had a good idea as to what it might be.

The family tree (*Figure 22*) confirmed my suspicions. Pointers to food allergies were there in abundance, for at least four generations.

Shirley herself was known to have had allergies to milk, eggs, peanuts and chocolate. Iris' maternal grandmother and uncle had asthma, which of course has well-established food allergy links. And Iris' mother had spent 40 years in a psychiatric hospital with puerperal psychosis, a psychosis that follows childbirth, and which, in every case I've ever investigated, accompanies a severe milk allergy. (The reason it normally appears after childbirth is that the new mother is told, "while you're breast-feeding you must drink lots of milk," with horrendous results if she's allergic to milk and normally doesn't drink it. Just think, if someone had thought to test Iris' mom for milk allergy during those 40 years, she might have been home in a few days.)

I was sure that food allergies would be revealed as Trevor and Trent's prime problem-causers. Tests quickly proved that to be the case. Trevor's test included yeast and several foods. Trent was allergic to yeast, malt, wheat, barley and egg white. In addition, his range of autoantibodies suggested he was well on the way to having celiac disease.

It was interesting, too, that Trent's father was also a psychiatric patient and had a known wheat allergy. The severity of Trent's symptoms could thus have been due to allergy-sensitive genes from both sides. In his mother's family, the sensitivity was being passed from mother to daughter and daughter to children in what looked to be an X-linked fashion. It's a safe bet that Iris has food allergies, too, and I'm testing her for them at the time of this writing.

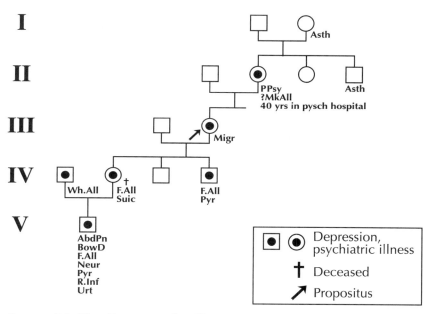

FIGURE 22: The Ransome family

A tragedy explained, and hope for the future: abundant pointers to food allergies for at least four generations.

Abd Pn	= Abdominal pain
Asth	= Asthma
Bow D	= Bowel disorders
F All	= Food allergies
Migr	= Migraine
?Mk All	= Milk Allergies?
Neur	= Neurasthenia (chronic lack of energy)
P Psy	= Puerperal psychosis
R Inf	= Recurring infections
Suic	= Suicide
Urt	= Urticaria (hives)
Wh All	= Wheat allergies

So, the Ransome family's apparently hereditary schizophrenia was actually a hypersensitivity to components
of their diet, which they were genetically unable to han-
dle. Trying to treat it with antidepressants or shock treatment might have touched the symptoms but would have
missed the cause. Lasting progress would only be made
when the food allergies were identified and a dietary
program established. I was able to do just that for Trevor
and Trent.

Trevor had actually been pretty well since his mother
had put him onto vitamins, but he was even better once
we got him off the foods which, through allergic reactions, were causing vitamin deficiencies.

Trent was the one who really benefited. To see that
pale, listless, infection-prone little boy turn into a normal, active kid with no bowel problems, and who
excelled at school, was one of those experiences that
makes you feel good to be a doctor. And best of all was
the knowledge that, thanks to the advance warning given
by his family tree, he should now avoid the family psychosis.

The family tree did two vital things for Trent. First,
it showed clearly that he was at risk for the schizophre-
nia-like illness. If left untreated, he almost certainly
would have developed it. Second, it showed us the real
nature of that illness, and what to do now to protect
Trent from it.

In addition, of course, the family tree cast a ray of
hope over future generations of Ransomes. From now on,
if anyone in the family develops psychiatric symptoms,
we know why. And we know what tests to do.

What's more, we can even predict which unborn
members of the family are most at risk. Trevor and Trent
both have faulty X chromosomes to pass on, so their
daughters will need to be watched, but not their sons.
However, Iris' other son, Geoff, is symptom-free, so
he apparently received a good X chromosome. Consequently, his children will all avoid the family problems.

It's surprising how many benefits can come from one family tree. It's still more surprising to me that so few doctors, particularly psychiatrists, use the family history as a diagnostic, therapeutic and predictive tool.

I hope this book will do something to change that.

THE TIME-MACHINE EFFECT: A SUMMARY

If you find an illness running through three or four generations of your family, try to work out how it's being transmitted – whether it's X-linked or autosomal, dominant or recessive. Use the examples given in Chapter 2 to help you here. It's not always easy to work out the mode of transmission, but quite often it is; and if you can pick it, you've achieved a major breakthrough.

When you know how the problem is being transmitted, you can see at a glance exactly who in your family is at risk for it, and who will dodge it completely.

Once again, the examples in Chapter 2 will help you to see that. But if you're not sure of the mode of transmission, and the problem is a serious one, play it safe. Find a doctor who understands the significance of family histories, and discuss the whole situation with him or her.

Frequently, as happened with the Woodbridge family, there will be genetic markers running along with the illness. These are usually, but not always, X-linked. If present, they are a tremendous help in working out whether you're at risk for a family illness. These markers can be conditions like color blindness, Xg blood grouping, or a tendency to prematurely gray hair. They can be hereditary food allergies or vitamin deficiencies. They can be physical characteristics like red hair, short stature, a prominent nose or buck teeth.

They become significant if you observe that, over two or three generations of your family, they occur in precisely the same people who have the particular illness you're tracking. This is a very good indication that the tendency for the illness is on the same chromosome as the marker. So, if you have that marker, whatever it may be, you're clearly at risk for the illness that has accompanied it in previous generations.

That doesn't mean that you'll automatically get it. It does mean that your risk for doing so is higher than the average – maybe just a little higher, maybe considerably higher. But forewarned is forearmed. Whether the illness is cancer, depression, schizophrenia, pernicious anemia, diabetes, multiple sclerosis or any of a dozen others, there are many preventative steps you can take. And you probably have years in which to take them. We'll look into that heartening fact in more detail in later chapters.

DENNIS: GOOD NEWS FROM GENETIC MARKERS

Of course, it isn't always bad news if you do share some genetic markers with an ancestor. It can, in fact, be very good news indeed – as I had the pleasure of informing a worried young man named Dennis.

He was a bright young fellow who had applied for a job in the public service. As anyone who has ever done that will know, it involves much filling out of forms. One question on the medical form probed into the applicant's family medical history – and immediately presented Dennis with a formidable hurdle. He had no health problems at all. His father, on the other hand, was a chronic paranoid schizophrenic. So was his mother, his maternal grandfather and his brother and sister. Dennis knew only too well that the public service people would be, to put it mildly, taken aback by a family history like that.

They were. In fact, it was almost certain that Dennis wouldn't be appointed to the permanent staff. He had a chance of making it as a casual, but that would mean very limited job prospects, and no chance of admittance to the splendid superannuation scheme.

However, before making the final decision, the public-service authorities sent Dennis to me for a *prognosis*. This was a polite way of saying, "If we appoint this guy, he'll go round the bend in a short space of time – right?"

Happily, after seeing Dennis and his family tree, I was able to answer, "Wrong."

How could I say that so confidently? True, Dennis himself was obviously quite sane. He was also remarkably well-adjusted, considering that he had spent all his family life with people subject to recurring mental illness. But, how could I tell that he wouldn't become a victim himself in the next few years?

Well – take a look at Dennis's family tree (*Figure 23*). The schizophrenic illness first showed up in Dennis's maternal grandfather. It moved down to his mother. It then came through to his brother and sister. Three generations – in a classic X-linked dominant pattern that was too clear-cut to be coincidental.

Dennis, however, shared no genetic markers with his brother, sister and maternal grandfather. His hair, eyes and complexion were all a different color from theirs. Significantly, they were very similar to those of his maternal uncle, who was also totally free of the schizophrenic illness. Dennis's brother and sister, on the other hand, were carbon copies of their grandfather, as regards hair, eyes and complexion color. The conclusion was obvious.

The grandfather had passed his faulty X chromosome on to Dennis's mother. Her other X chromosome, obtained from her healthy mother, had been normal. But because the faulty one was dominant, the illness appeared in her. Her brother (Dennis's uncle) didn't, of course, get their father's faulty X chromosome. He received his X chromosome from his mother, as sons always do. It was a normal one, so he was free of the illness.

Dennis's mother, then, had one faulty and one normal chromosome. In the genetic lottery, Dennis's brother and sister both received the faulty one. Dennis received the normal one. So, like his uncle and grandmother before him, he was at no risk whatsoever for the family illness.

But what about the genetic influence of his schizophrenic father?

I couldn't see any worries there, either. The clue was Dennis's sister. She, poor girl, was the worst affected of the whole family – and the logical explanation for that was that she had inherited not only her mother's faulty X chromosome, but a similar one from her father as well. That, in turn, suggested that the father's problem was

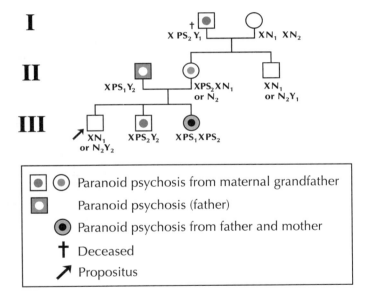

FIGURE 23: Dennis

Good news – and a new career – from a family tree.

Y_1 = Y chromosome from maternal grandfather
Y_2 = Y chromosome from father
XN_1 = Normal chromosome not at risk for paranoid psychosis
XN_2 = Normal chromosome not at risk for paranoid psychosis
XPS_1 = X chromosome from father with gene for paranoid psychosis
XPS_2 = X chromosome from maternal grandfather with gene for paranoid psychosis

X-linked – which of course meant that he couldn't pass it on to Dennis. Therefore, Dennis was quite safe from that side too.

When I explained all this on Dennis's report, the public-service authorities accepted it. Dennis was taken onto the permanent staff – thanks to the genetic markers on his family tree, which pointed to a totally normal future for him.

It was good to be able to help Dennis in that way. But I couldn't help regretting that he and his family weren't my patients. I'm sure I could have really helped his brother and sister by identifying the X-linked condition that was causing the family's psychotic illness.

It could have been X-linked food allergies, leading to vitamin deficiencies, especially B_6, B_{12} or B_3. Or an X-linked immunoglobulin disturbance. Or an X-linked enzyme defect. Or any of a dozen other things. But, whatever it was, the principle we outlined in the last chapter would have applied. Find the associated X-linked metabolic defect, treat it, and you'll treat the problem.

In Dennis's case, the family tree's time-machine effect revealed that he had a genetically sound future. And, of course, it could look a lot further down the track than that. If Dennis had children, for instance, they would not be at any risk for the X-linked family illness, because Dennis had no faulty chromosomes to pass on.

That wouldn't be the case, however, with his brother and sister. All the sister's sons and daughters would invariably get it, because both her X chromosomes contained a faulty dominant gene. The brother's sons would be safe, but all his daughters would become victims. So, you could tell who was at risk in the next generation, and further, as long as the faulty genes persisted.

Incidentally, I happened to meet Dennis, by chance, in the street about five years later. He was in excellent health, enjoying his job, and starting to climb up the public-service ladder – thanks to his family tree, without which he wouldn't have made the first rung.

LOOKING BACKWARDS . . . AND SIDEWAYS

As well as peering into the future, family trees can frequently also take a beneficial look backwards . . . or sideways.

Families like the Ransomes and Woodbridges often have relatives, elderly or not so elderly, tucked away in psychiatric wards. Doctors have assumed, perhaps for years, that these folk are chronic schizophrenics for whom nothing can be done. But if it's established that other family members have psychoses due to food allergies, celiac disease, vitamin deficiencies, anemia or SLE, then there's new hope for these apparently hopeless people. I've seen patients, who have spent many years in a hospital, go home in a month once a family tree has suggested the real cause of their illness.

A family tree can also set minds at rest – or sow a salutary seed of disquiet where none existed before.

JACK'S MOTHER HAZEL: A FEAR REMOVED

Hark back for a moment to Jack's family tree (*Figure 21*). We've looked thoroughly at Jack's problems, and those waiting around the corner for his children. Now let's consider Jack's mother, Hazel, who for some time had lived under a cloud of dread.

Her white blood cell count was at a very low level and there were changes taking place in the structure of her bone marrow. Taken together, those two conditions suggested the development of benign myeloid leukemia. That in itself was not too serious – benign myeloid leukemia can smolder away for years without you even realizing that you have it. But, for Hazel, it was very disconcerting indeed. After all, her brother had died of acute leukemia. Her mother had died of Hodgkin's disease, which, like leukemia, is a form of cancer. Her uncle and aunt had both died of pernicious anemia, another blood disorder that in those days was frequently fatal.

Was she to be the next in the list of fatalities?

It was a totally understandable fear. And, it was very rewarding to be able to put her mind at rest. You'll remember that she, like Jack and his daughters, had severe grain allergies. These seemed to be autosomal dominant in transmission. Consequently, Hazel's mother, brother, uncle and aunt almost certainly had them, too. And grain allergies are known to be linked with the very illnesses that killed them – leukemia, Hodgkin's disease and pernicious anemia. So it was overwhelmingly likely that those problems were primarily caused by the family's grain allergies.

That had major implications for Hazel. It meant that the development of leukemia changes in her blood was not a mysterious or inevitable process. It was, in all probability, a direct result of her grain allergy. Therefore, if she strictly avoided grains, the problem could be expected to go away.

And it did. Some months after she went on a grain-free diet, a blood test showed a marked improvement in her white cell count.

The chances of her getting acute leukemia had drastically diminished – and a great weight had been lifted from her mind.

JACK'S BROTHER TED: A WARNING MESSAGE

But, while the family tree was setting her mind at ease, it was pointing a disquieting finger elsewhere. At Jack's brother, Ted, who suffered from chronic sinusitis and hay fever. And at Ted's little daughter, Megan, a very quiet, shy girl with infantile eczema and asthma.

Allergic complaints, all of them. Not to be wondered at, in a family like Jack's – but were they tip-of-the-iceberg indicators of more serious conditions underneath? Were the family's grain allergies, at work in both Ted and Megan, paving the way for future cancers, leukemias, pernicious anemia and psychiatric problems?

The possibility was quite high, given the grain allergies' probable autosomal dominant mode of transmission. If Ted and Megan had been my patients, I would have strongly recommended the appropriate tests. I would have emphasized that the opportunity to identify, and head off, major problems years before they arose was just too good to miss.

But I wasn't their doctor, so I couldn't. All I could do was pass on a message through Jack – a message explaining what the family tree's time-machine function had done for Jack's children, and what it could very well do for Ted and Megan.

Perhaps your family tree can do as much, if not more, for you. And the other person it can really help is your doctor; because, as we've seen in these last three chapters, it can help him to do a far better job of looking after you.

Wouldn't you like him to be able to diagnose your problems with new accuracy? To know immediately what tests to do? To see more quickly the right course of treatment? To tell you what illnesses you and your children are most at risk for – and to take positive steps to guard you against them?

Well, you can help your doctor to do all those things. Give him a really good, comprehensive family tree and insist that he (or she) look for the warning signs.

PART TWO

Your Family Tree: How to Compile It and What It Can Tell You

We've seen what family trees are doing for other people. Now it's time to consider what yours can do for you. We'll start this section by learning how to draw up your family tree, what to put on it and where to find that information.

Then we'll consider what the information means – and how you can use your family tree to protect you and your family from a host of unpleasant diseases. You may be in the firing line for some kind of hereditary problem, but that doesn't mean you have to stand there and let it get you.

In most cases, there's a great deal you can do to avoid it. This section tells you how.

⁘6⁘

How to Draw up Your Family Tree

There is, of course, one thing you have to do before you can give your doctor a brilliantly informative family tree – you have to draw it up.

To do so, you obviously need to know what conditions to include and how to include them. It also helps the doctor to read it if you lay it out properly and use the right symbols. So, we'll learn to do all that now, before we take a further look at some of the growing evidence for the medical value of family trees.

THE BASIC FAMILY TREE

The first step is to lay out the basic framework for as many generations as you are able to go back. Let's look (*Figure 24*) at a very simple, hypothetical family tree of four generations (most people can, with a little research, go back at least that far).

From this simple diagram, note the following points:

- males are represented by squares, and females by circles;
- each generation is on a separate line;
- the generations are numbered downwards in Roman numerals;
- the people in each generation are numbered from left to right in normal (Arabic) numerals;
- the person being considered (called – ready for it – the proband or *propositus*) is indicated by an arrow.
- Everyone else is then known by their relationship to him or her (e.g., father, maternal aunt, paternal cousin, etc.).

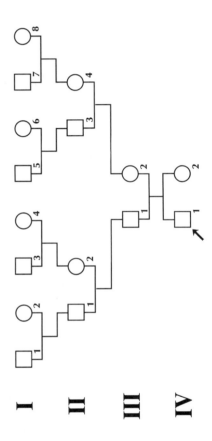

FIGURE 24: the basic family tree

A hypothetical four-generation sample that shows the basic principles of drawing up a family tree

Naturally, like a tree, a family tree gets wider as it goes up, due to the indisputable fact that everyone has two parents, four grandparents, eight great-grand-parents, and so on.

THE EXPANDED FAMILY TREE

OK so far? Right. Now let's take that same diagram, and add in some aunts, uncles, cousins, twins, stillbirths, miscarriages, adopted children, second marriages and deaths (*Figure 25*).

That's made it look a lot more complicated, but it's not really (and few families would have all that happening in four generations, anyway). The points to note here are:

- aunts, uncles and cousins must be kept in their right generations (they have a way of creeping up or down a line, which thoroughly confuses the whole picture);
- twins are indicated by squares or circles, springing from a common point, and labeled "I" for identical twins, "F" for fraternal twins;
- stillbirths and miscarriages are indicated by small black squares or circles if the sex is known, or small triangles if it isn't;
- adopted children are distinguished by a broken vertical line, with two short horizontal lines through it;
- second marriages are indicated by a second line that runs down from the person concerned, then across and up to the second partner, on the opposite side of the person from the first partner;
- deaths are shown by a cross, with the age at death in figures, beside the person's symbol.

Still with me? If so, you've grasped all the basic rules needed to lay out your family tree. Now we get to the meat of it – what to put on the family tree, and why.

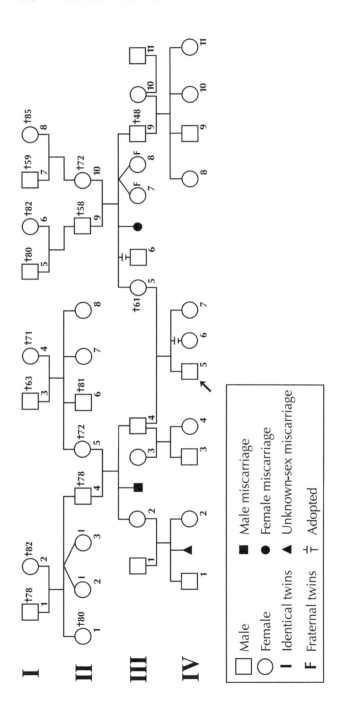

FIGURE 25: the expanded family tree

It looks more complicated, but the basic principles still apply.

I've found that it's a good idea to start by writing down all possible information about each person on a separate sheet of paper. From that list, you then select what will actually go on the family tree. That's much easier and neater than writing everything straight onto your framework, and perhaps having to cross out things or alter them later on.

START WITH DIAGNOSED ILLNESSES

Basically, of course, what we're after is medical information. So the first thing for your list is actual diagnosed illnesses and conditions. I don't mean that you put on every individual cold or bout of flu; but, you do include illnesses of a chronic or recurring nature, as well as the obviously serious and fatal ones.

For instance, you would include colds and flu if they occurred on an unusually regular basis. This would indicate that the person was subject to recurring infections, which could be a vital piece of information.

One thing you may well notice is that the illnesses in your family tend to fall into categories. That is, you'll find several people all suffering from heart and blood vessel disorders. Or glandular problems. Or cancer. Or psychiatric illnesses. And so on.

If you do, that will, of course, be very significant. It will show that a genetic predisposition for those illnesses is indeed running through your family. What's more, by tracing its course through the generations, you will probably be able to tell its mode of transmission – whether X-linked dominant, X-linked recessive, autosomal dominant, or otherwise. And, as we've seen previously, you can then tell who is in the firing line, in this and future generations.

Two questions, I suspect, have leaped into your mind. How can you tell which illnesses should be grouped together into a category? (What, for instance, are glandular problems?) And if one relative had 12 things wrong with her, how can you fit them all onto one family tree?

The answer to the first question is in Appendix A at the back of the book. There you'll find a list of illnesses, all neatly gathered into their respective categories. It's not an exhaustive inventory of all known human ills, but it does include the most likely ones.

The answer to the second question is simple: you don't try. If you do find a great batch of diseases running through the family, you start by categorizing them. Then you prepare a separate family tree for each category: heart and blood vessel disorders, cancers, neurological: problems, respiratory illnesses, and so on.

The benefits of that are twofold. First of all, it's easier for you, and it enables you to fit everything in. Second, it shows your doctor the significant patterns right away. He or she doesn't have to untangle them from a mass of information. They're clearly revealed, and obvious at a glance.

As you've doubtless noticed from the family trees so far, the illnesses on each are listed by means of an abbreviation. This is a practical way of putting them on (imagine trying to fit *systemic lupus erythematosus* into your diagram). After you've learned that a particular relative had a particular illness, just locate that illness in the table, note its category and give it a simple abbreviation. That abbreviation then goes next to the person's symbol on your finished family tree. If you're doing a separate family tree for each of several categories of illness, you have to make sure, of course, that it's on the right one.

After you've put all your abbreviations into place, here's an important tip. List them all somewhere on the bottom of your family tree, together with the full names of the illnesses they represent. That will ensure that you and your doctor are on the same abbreviation wavelength (if you put "PLS" meaning *pyloric stenosis*, and he or she interprets it as "piles," your family tree's message will, to put it mildly, be obscured).

THE FAMILY TREE PLUS ILLNESSES

Having absorbed all that, we'll now see how our hypothetical family tree looks with some illnesses added in
(*Figure 26*). We'll take out the stillbirths, adoptions, second marriages and so on for simplicity's sake, remove one
lot of great-grandparents, add some more aunts and
uncles, and make it a family tree of heart and blood
vessel disorders.

As it stands now, this is modeled fairly closely on a
real family tree from my files. Can you tell how the heart
and blood vessel problems are being transmitted – and
the people who are at risk for developing them?

If you said *X-linked* dominant, and named children 4,
5, 7, 10 and 11 in generation IV as being at risk, you're
right on. Note how the abbreviations are used, and how
they are listed and explained at the bottom.

So that's how known, diagnosed illnesses go into your
family tree. It's a pretty straightforward business – as long
as you're aware of, or can discover, the actual illnesses
that have punctuated your family's history.

ADDING SYMPTOMS AND SIGNS

But what if many illnesses, perhaps in key relatives or forebears, have never been diagnosed? It often happens that,
while family members may have had plenty of things
wrong with them, no one actually got around to labeling
their aches, pains and general woes. What then? Are
you prevented from drawing up a medically significant
family tree?

No, you're not. You mightn't be able to name all the
actual illnesses, but you may still be able to draw up an
excellent family tree of symptoms and signs. To an alert
doctor, that may be quite enough for some specific
diagnoses, which could then point clearly to the troublemakers in your family's genetic inheritance.

Even if you can compile some good family trees in various illness categories, you may find several interesting

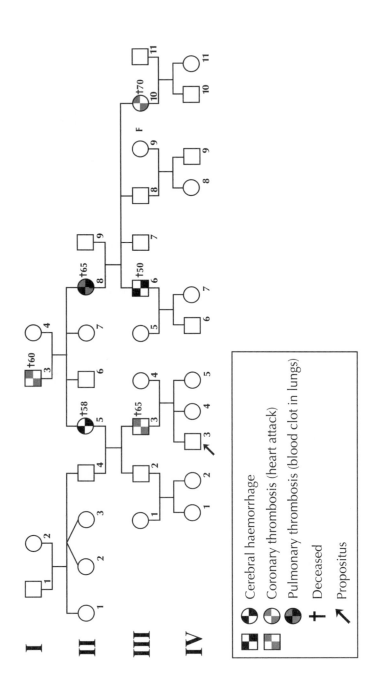

FIGURE 26: the family tree with illnesses added
Our hypothetical family tree purged of some excess relatives, with heart and blood vessel disorders added.

symptoms and signs in the family as well. In that case, unless they obviously belong in one category or another, it's still worth doing an extra family tree with only them on it. Such a *symptoms-and-signs* family tree could provide just the extra clue needed to tie the whole picture together.

What, you ask, do we mean precisely by *symptoms-and-signs*? Basically, a "symptom" is something you *feel* (like headaches, tiredness or nausea), while a "sign" is something that another person can *observe* (like premature gray hair, cracks around the corners of the mouth or obesity).

The amount of genetic light they can shed on a family tree is quite surprising – especially when they are linked with known diagnoses in other family members, when they occur in several people, or when two or more of them go together.

For example, say you had a few people in the family who complained of chronic fatigue (not an illness, but a symptom). On its own, that could mean almost anything. But, if you had some others with diabetes, the chances would be quite high that the fatigue sufferers also had diabetes, or were developing it. If they had linked conditions, such as cataracts or a leg amputation as well, the chances would escalate to a near certainty.

You would then know two important things. First, you would know, with some degree of assurance, what was actually wrong with the fatigued people, past or present. Second, you would have a much clearer picture of how the tendency toward diabetes was being transmitted through your family – and who needed to take precautions against it.

Of course, you mightn't have known that chronic fatigue, cataracts and the need for leg amputation are linked with diabetes. Or which other symptoms and signs go with which diseases. But, to your doctor, who does know, a *symptoms-and-signs* family tree could be a vital diagnostic breakthrough. That's why it's so worthwhile to compile one – even if you also have some detailed family trees in one or more categories of illness.

The number of symptoms and signs that family members could have observed in each other, or remember older relatives talking about, is almost limitless. But if any of the following have occurred in your family on a regular basis, it's worth including them on a family tree:

- headaches, migraine, blackouts, fainting spells, convulsions;
- weakness, lassitude, chronic tiredness or lack of energy – especially if linked with premature deafness, overweight, depression, double vision, loss of coordination, slurred voice, cataracts, need for amputations (gangrene), boils;
- mouth ulcers or sores, cold sores, cracks around corners of mouth, sores on the tongue;
- premature hair loss, prematurely gray hair, patches of white skin (depigmented areas);
- depression, mood swings, extreme activity, non-stop or excessive talking, poor memory, inability to concentrate;
- changes in color or shape or texture of fingernails, toenails or skin, easy bruising;
- abdominal pain, nausea, flatulence (increased "wind"), bowel frequency or regular diarrhea, indigestion – especially in people who are overweight or underweight;
- food cravings, whether in pregnancy or not – "sweet tooth," headaches or nausea if meals are missed, craving for salt, ice, milk, cheese, yeast extracts, bananas, pickles, tomatoes, oranges, lettuce, etc., cravings for bizarre things like soil or clay (pica).

Even this list is by no means exhaustive. If you turn to Appendix B, you'll find a much more complete list of potentially significant symptoms and signs, including a group of psychiatric ones.

What do they all mean? Many are explained in detail in Chapters 7 to 10. To your doctor, the significance of all of them for you and your family should be readily apparent.

A *SYMPTOMS-AND-SIGNS* FAMILY TREE

Let's see exactly what a family tree of symptoms and signs might look like, and what it might reveal (*Figure 27*).

This hypothetical example contains some pretty common symptoms and signs. Taken individually, they wouldn't say much to anyone; but linked together in these combinations and successions, they would immediately alert any savvy doctor to the presence of

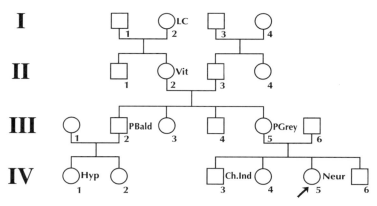

FIGURE 27: symptoms and signs

A number of conditions that don't mean much on their own, but speak volumes when gathered onto a family tree.

Ch Ind   = Chronic indigestion
Hyp   = Hyperactivity
L C   = Leg cramps
Neur   = Neurasthenia (chronic lack of energy)
P Bald   = Premature baldness
P Gray   = Premature graying
Vit   = Vitiligo (patches of white skin)

X-linked food allergies, with consequent vitamin and mineral deficiencies. They would be like an arrow pointing in the direction of diagnosis, treatment and future prevention.

So, now we know how to draw up the family tree and how to put illnesses on it. We also know about such refinements as separate family trees for various categories of illnesses, and the diagnostic potential of symptoms and signs.

If we left it at that, you could certainly compile a family tree of enormous medical value to you and your children. But if you're prepared to put a little more time and effort into it, there's a whole host of extra things you can add – and I think the additional trouble is very well worth taking.

After all, while it's good to know what illnesses are running in your family, it's even better to know what's causing them. That can often be discovered from the basic information I've already suggested, but some extra data would definitely make the job easier. It would make your family tree even more medically valuable in other ways, and perhaps give it real research importance as well.

CONGENITAL ABNORMALITIES

The first of these *extra* categories would be the presence in your family tree of any congenital conditions or abnormalities.

Congenital simply means "present at birth." While the term could, by definition, be applied to happy and beneficial things, in practice it's usually reserved for the problems and disabilities with which a person is born. Examples include deformities such as clubfoot, cleft palate and harelip, crippling conditions such as spina bifida and cerebral palsy (spasticity), and congenital illnesses like cystic fibrosis and certain heart ailments.

If any such things have occurred in your family, it's worth putting them on your family tree. By themselves, they can be important pointers to conditions that are running in your family. They can confirm a tentative diagnosis, or even suggest one. In addition, they often have great value as genetic markers. That is to say, they can help you to see how a condition is being transmitted through your family and, consequently who is at risk for it.

For instance, red-green color blindness (an important congenital abnormality) is known to be transmitted in an X-linked way. Suppose that several people in your family were red-green color-blind, or were carriers of the trait, and those same people all had a particular illness – say, pernicious anemia. You'd immediately suspect that the pernicious anemia was being transmitted genetically. And on the same X chromosome as the color blindness.

Consequently, if you also happened to be red-green color-blind, you would be at real risk for the pernicious anemia. The genetic marker would be pointing ominously at you – but in time for you to do something about it.

True, not all congenital abnormalities have such genetic significance. Cerebral palsy, for instance, is often caused by a birth accident. When it is, it's no more meaningful in your family tree than a sprained ankle. So, if you're certain that congenital abnormalities have been caused by birth accidents, don't include them. But, if you're not sure, put them in – and let your doctor decide.

These are only a few examples of congenital abnormalities; you'll find a list of the more common ones in Appendix C.

PHENOTYPES

There's another set of congenital conditions that can add a lot to a family tree's value. While they're *not exactly* abnormalities and don't always involve factors that are a little out of the ordinary, *sometimes* they do. I'm referring here to anything uncommon or distinctive about one's physical appearance; especially in the areas of unusual height (tallness or shortness), weight or general physical type.

Such characteristics are important for two reasons. First, they sometimes make excellent genetic markers. And genetic markers, as we saw a moment ago, are very valuable indeed. In fact, when you set out to plot the path of disease through your family, you can't have too many of them.

It's worth restating: if a genetic marker coincides with a particular illness in several people over a few generations and, if that same marker is present in you, then you have a warning of your risk for that illness, years in advance. Which you certainly wouldn't have without your family tree.

Second, unusual physical types or *phenotypes*, to use the technical term, can be a lot more than genetic markers. They can actually be valuable diagnostic aids. In recent years, the fascinating fact has emerged that some physical types are clearly linked with certain medical conditions and personality traits.

There is, for instance, what is known as the *Pyknic* build – a short, stocky physique, often with an unusually broad forehead. This is definitely associated with manic-depressive illness. So, if the problem in your family were swings of mood, and if there were, or had been, family members with that sort of build, you'd think of manic-depressive illness right away. And those people's position in your family tree would tell you two other things – how the illness, or its cause, was being transmitted through your family, and who was next in line.

Another telltale physical type is the exact opposite of the Pyknic build. Known as the *Marfan Syndrome*, it produces people who are unusually tall and thin. They have long spindly fingers, and are particularly prone to three physical defects: a lens problem in the eye, high blood pressure and thrombosis, and serious heart problems. The heart problems frequently start with a narrowing of the aorta, the main heart artery. This, in turn, tends to cause an aneurysm (a ballooning), or even a fatal rupture, of the artery wall.

Doctors are pretty sure now that Abraham Lincoln was a classic example of the Marfan Syndrome; and that his heart problems could well have lowered a premature curtain on his career, even if John Wilkes Booth had not visited the theatre on that fateful night.

The Marfan Syndrome is transmitted in an autosomal dominant way. That means, as you'll remember, that it appears in roughly half the children, male and female, of those who have it. And not at all in the direct descendants of those who don't.

As a result, it's not too hard to pick out in a family tree. If you've had people in your family with eye and heart defects, and who were also abnormally tall and thin, put them down and check how the conditions are being transmitted. If it looks like an autosomal dominant picture, the Marfan Syndrome could well be your problem.

But even if it were, would you be any better off for knowing it?

Yes, you would be. You would know that the family's eye, blood pressure and heart problems were not savagely random things, but were predictable – because they were part of a condition being transmitted in an autosomal dominant way. And you would then know exactly who, in this and future generations, needed to have regular checks for eye problems, high blood pressure and heart disease. Checks that could not only save their sight, but also their lives.

There's also another possibility: You could have tall, thin people with heart and eye problems in your family tree who aren't linked together in an autosomal dominant way.

That, too, would be very significant. To the alert doctor, it would immediately suggest a condition called *homocystinuria*, which is a kind of first cousin to the Marfan Syndrome. While it produces the same kind of effects, it is really a much more amiable member of the family, for two important reasons. First, it is autosomal recessive in transmission, so it bobs up in considerably fewer people. Second, in some cases, it responds very well to Vitamin B_6 treatment. So once you've identified it, something can often be done about it right away.

Consequently, if tall, thin sufferers of heart and eye complaints were scattered through your family in an autosomal recessive pattern, your family tree would perform all three of its vital roles in one swoop.

To your alert doctor, it would make the diagnosis and line of treatment for present sufferers as plain as a pikestaff. It would also identify those at risk in the future. The vital factor in enabling it to do that? Simply, that you'd added a tall, thin physique to the information about heart and eye problems in your family tree. So you can see how important any details of unusual phenotypes can be.

A few years ago, interest in phenotypes reached a new height when some researchers claimed that all human beings could be separated into three categories. Further, they claimed that each of these phenotypes had its own typical personality traits.

The three types were named ectomorphs, endomorphs and mesomorphs. Ectomorphs, the theory ran, are the tall, thin, lightly muscled people who tend to be introverted and bookish. Endomorphs are those solidly built folk with hearty, extrovert, hail-fellow-well-met kinds of personalities. And mesomorphs are the rugged, muscular types who excel in the physical and sporting areas of life.

Personally, keen fan of phenotypes though I am, I was never too sold on this particular theory. And I'm interested to see that more and more experts are sharing my skepticism. It's true that I know more people, and probably you do too, who fit perfectly into one or other of the categories. It's also true that the theory's proponents add that each of us is something of a mixture of all three types.

Nevertheless, I've met too many tall, thin people who are fiercely extroverted and achievement-oriented. I've met too many solidly built folk who are shy and introverted to the point of total withdrawal. And I've met too many rugged, muscular people whose greatest athletic achievement is to raise a cold beer can to their parched lips.

No, it's an attractive theory, but I think human personality is a little more complex than that. The kind of phenotypes that I find useful in a family tree are those that occur in definite association with medical or psychiatric conditions, symptoms and signs.

OTHER TELLTALE PHYSICAL SIGNS

Several other kinds of physical appearance, while not exactly phenotypes because you're not actually born with them, can be valuable diagnostic aids – hence, well worth recording in your family tree. For instance, does your family contain people who are thin, with protruding eyes, and who also tend to be nervous and anxious? The combination is very frequently linked with an overactive thyroid.

Conversely, do you have people who are overweight with sallow complexions, and the unusual feature of hair loss on the outer third of the eyebrows? That's a strong indication of the opposite problem – an underactive thyroid – especially if those folk also become deaf and develop hoarse voices.

Overactive or underactive thyroids are often missed by doctors – yet they are responsible for a multitude of unpleasant physical and psychiatric effects. Even if their external clues don't appear in the current generation, their presence in previous ones would be very significant. They would certainly point to thyroid disorders running in the family and, in all probability, unmask them as the underlying cause of the current generation's problems.

The inclusion of lots of other physical characteristics can be equally valuable. If your family has members with very broad foreheads, fair complexions and prematurely gray hair, you probably have pernicious anemia (a massive Vitamin B_{12} deficiency) running through your ranks. It responds well to large doses of Vitamin B_{12}.

Or, if you have some short people with smallish head circumference, you can suspect that celiac disease has stunted their growth. And you can look for spectacular improvement once the celiac disease (an allergy to components of grain, such as gluten) has been considered, diagnosed and treated. A dramatic example was little Kevin, a short, runty child from just such a family. Kevin loved swimming, but he could swim only a few yards when I first saw him. After a year's treatment for celiac disease, he had grown several inches taller, and gone from last in his school class to first. He was also Australian swimming champion for his age group.

James's experience was almost as dramatic. He was three years old, but had the physique of a one-year-old. He was so small and weak that he couldn't even support himself or crawl. Once again, the family tree suggested celiac disease. Treatment began, and over the next year James grew normally. He was walking unaided shortly after his fourth birthday.

All because, in both instances, short stature and small head size were included in the family tree.

Another recurring pattern in some families is people who are of average height, but unusually thin. This suggests that milk and grain allergies are preventing them from absorbing all the nutrients in their food. Consequently, a family tree full of skinny people always prompts me to check for milk and grain allergies, and I've rarely been wrong on that score.

A related, but rather rare, pattern is the one where people are quite literally a different size from day to day. They have a thing called *Osler's Syndrome* (*hereditary angioedema*), an extreme sensitivity to certain foods, chemicals and pollens. When an *Osler's Syndrome* sufferer comes into contact with any of those substances, his or her limbs, body and face swell up – so much so, that I've known people who have to keep several sizes of clothes to cope with the problem. This makes the illness not only uncomfortable and embarrassing, but also expensive.

Osler's Syndrome is transmitted in an autosomal dominant way. When you see this relationship among people whose bodies regularly swell up, you know what you're up against. Tests can then identify the offending substances. By avoiding them, the patient gains relief, and substantially lowers clothing bills.

Physical appearance is also the clue to another autosomal dominant condition – one that bears the majestic title of *von Recklinghausen's Syndrome* or *neurofibromatosis*. The distinctive feature is lots of lumps and nodules distributed all over the patient's face and body. Pigmented areas of skin, known as cafe-au-lait spots, often occur with them. The significance of the whole unpleasant syndrome is that it is very frequently associated with brain and spinal cord tumors.

Consequently, if this readily recognized syndrome is in your family tree, you can easily work out whether or not you're in the autosomal dominant firing line. If you are, you should have regular checkups for brain and spinal cord tumors – even if you don't have the lumps, spots and nodules; and especially if you notice any unusual nausea; disturbances of vision, speech and muscular coordination; weakness in the legs; backaches or loss of sensation in the legs or back. The earlier these tumors are diagnosed, the more chance you have of beating them.

Superficially similar to von Recklinghausen's Syndrome, but actually quite different, is *Dercum's disease*. It also produces lumps all over the body, which on closer examination turn out to be fatty cysts. Dercum's disease is autosomal recessive in transmission and well worth recording in a family tree: sneaking along with it is the increased risk of heart disease – another area where early warnings carry with them the seeds of victory.

Several other illnesses are, like Dercum's disease, active in the business of dumping fatty lumps and deposits about the body. Typical of them is one that rejoices in the name of *hereditary hypercholesterolemia* (and, would you believe, that's one of the simpler names of illnesses in this category).

In the case of this particular tongue twister, the visible lumps are little yellowish plaques of fat known as xanthelasma. These appear below the eyelids and between the corner of the eye and the nose. Also visible in some sufferers is a white circle around the iris of the eye. This is known as arcus senilis, and is usually confined to elderly people. When it occurs in younger folk and children – especially in those with xanthelasma around the eyes and nose – it is a good pointer to hereditary hypercholesterolemia.

Autosomal dominant in transmission, hereditary hypercholesterolemia is accompanied by a high risk for arteriosclerosis – the development inside arteries of fatty deposits that severely restrict blood flow. Arteriosclerosis is a prime cause of heart attacks, kidney disorders, brain damage and many other unpleasant events.

So the telltale outward signs of hereditary hypercholesterolemia are certainly worth mentioning in a family tree. They can explain why lots of nasty things have been happening in a family, and point to those next in line for them. More happily, they can also suggest preventable dietary reforms and other protective measures.

Height, weight, lumps and nodules aren't all that there is to physical appearance. The outward sign of a condition called *discoid lupus* involves none of those things – but is every bit as distinctive. It's found on the face, in the form of a bright red rash that covers both cheeks and tapers in toward the nose. Because of its shape, this is known as a butterfly rash. If you have people in your family, past or present, with this very noticeable feature, you'll probably have certain other conditions running through the family too.

Conditions such as arthritis, hair loss, mouth ulcers, migraine and photosensitivity (the tendency to burn easily in the sun). Chances are that there'll also be people who have had a stroke, perhaps a fatal one, or developed senile dementia. All these things combine with the outward sign of the butterfly rash to confirm the discoid lupus diagnosis. And, discoid lupus is closely associated with SLE, the connective tissue disorder that we've met several times in previous chapters. SLE, you'll remember, leads to psychiatric symptoms. Consequently, if there are people in your family with mental or emotional disorders, and if the red butterfly rash is there as well – whether on those same people or others – SLE is what you'd think of first. Especially if the other symptoms are also dogging the family's footsteps.

Discoid lupus is certainly transmitted genetically, although we're not quite sure of the exact form of transmission. It has been worked out that children of an affected mother have a 20 percent chance of getting it too.

By now, I think I've made the point that the extra step of adding phenotypes, physical characteristics and outward appearances to your family tree is well worth taking. Their presence in the current or previous generations can identify a whole host of glandular problems, allergic conditions, malabsorption states (those in which the body isn't properly absorbing nourishment), metabolic disorders and other ills that are notoriously hard to diagnose.

And, of course, once you identify the enemy, you know how to go about fighting him. To help you do this, you'll find a much more complete list of physical characteristics, appearance traits, phenotypes, and more, at the end of the book in Appendix D.

EPIDEMIOLOGICAL INFORMATION

One last category of *extras*, and I think we've covered all the information your family tree can hold. This one may sound exotic indeed; but, as we'll discover, solid benefits can flow from it, not only in the medical information field, but in the areas of research and sheer family interest as well.

This category covers what is learnedly called *epidemiological* information. That mouthful includes such things as ethnic background, lifestyle, environmental factors, religion, occupation and any unusual achievements in life – such as becoming a head of state or a convicted bank robber.

Let's start with the ethnic bit first. And I can hear your question now: what possible relevance can such information have in a family tree, the prime purpose of which is to forecast, diagnose, treat and prevent illness in your family? Surprisingly, a great deal.

For instance, did you know that certain illnesses occur more frequently in people of a particular nationality? They do, and it's a documented fact that I find quite fascinating.

To begin with, there's a higher-than-usual incidence of glucose-6-phosphate deficiency, leading to hereditary anemias, in Mediterranean and African people. (The sickle cell anemia that affects many black Americans, yet rarely appears in whites, is a well-known example.)

Congenital kidney disorders appear in an above-average rate among Finnish people. The incidence of stomach cancer in Japan is well above the global norm. A familial Mediterranean fever occurs most frequently in Armenian people. If you were born in Hawaii of Polynesian parents, you run a higher-than-average risk for clubfoot, diabetes and coronary heart disease.

And (dare I mention it?) the rate of major central nervous system malformation is highest among the Irish.

On the positive side, there are medical advantages running alongside the problems in some of these ethnic groups.

The Mediterranean people's risk for hereditary anemias is balanced by their unusually low incidence of cystic fibrosis. The Africans, too, are markedly low in cystic fibrosis, and also have less multiple sclerosis and hemophilia than other ethnic groups. The Armenians, despite their familial Mediterranean fever tendencies, have below-average rates of the glucose 6-phosphate deficiencies that worry the Mediterranean and African folk.

Fascinating, as I remarked before: but why is it so? That, I'm afraid, is the $64,000 question. Some authorities put it down to mutations in the gene pool that happened when each ethnic group was virtually self-contained. Others feel that local environmental factors, such as diet or soil and water content, are responsible.

Personally, I lean towards the first view, in certain cases at least. I've seen some of these typically ethnic conditions persist in a family despite generations of geographic relocation: which is why I think it's good to include ethnic origins in a family tree. In those instances, they point to a genetic factor in the family's illnesses, and so make a real contribution to diagnosis, prediction and prevention.

On the other hand, some epidemiological information helps in precisely the opposite way – by showing that certain family illnesses probably aren't genetic in origin, but are due to environmental factors. Information about the family's physical environment can reveal this. And it's important in a family tree for two reasons.

First, by revealing nongenetic factors in recurring family illness, it saves you from a fruitless search for non-existent genetic modes of transmission. That, in turn, prevents the danger of predicting the illness in someone who's not at risk or, worse, predicting the safety of someone who's very much at risk.

Second, if more and more people record both environmental factors and illnesses in family trees, I believe more and more evidence will emerge of links between the two. That clearly has tremendous value for research into the causes of all kinds of diseases.

Let me quote some examples.

No less than 46 percent of multiple sclerosis patients observed in a recent study had mothers who drank tank water (from rainwater run-off) while pregnant with them. Tank water is low in essential trace elements and minerals. What did the lack of those items do to the developing fetuses? Did it somehow predispose them to developing MS in the future? If so, how?

A Chinese study has shown a higher incidence of cancer of the esophagus (the food tube between throat and stomach) in areas where the soil was deficient in certain trace elements. The higher incidence applied both to people and animals. Chinese scientists deduced that the soil deficiency was lowering the ability of food plants to trap Vitamin C. They corrected the deficiency by fertilizing vast tracts of the area with molybdenum.

The startling result? The local incidence of esophageal cancer swiftly fell to normal levels. What does that suggest about a link between Vitamin C deficiencies and cancer?

In America, it was noted that people living around a new chemical processing plant were showing an above-average rate of cancer and congenital abnormalities. Tests showed that the soil was full of chemicals, especially mercury, which was being absorbed by local crops. That helped to confirm the already suspected role of certain chemicals in birth deformities and the development of cancer.

Strict members of the Seventh-Day Adventist Church don't eat meat. Studies have demonstrated that they live longer than the community norm, but that they also have a higher-than-average rate of pernicious anemia. Consequently, if a family tree contains cases of pernicious anemia, but also notes that the sufferers were strict Seventh-Day Adventists and vegetarians, then you would suspect an environmental cause rather than a genetic one.

You would do likewise if your relatives and forebears with cancer lived near chemical processing plants or in areas of known soil deficiencies, or were heavy smokers. The same deduction would apply to relatives with MS, if their mothers had lived on tank water during pregnancy.

In all those cases, the environmental information would keep you from drawing the wrong conclusions about the causes of family illness. It would also, incidentally, make your family tree into a valuable research document.

Of course, in many instances an environmental factor can cause problems because of a family genetic trait. Remember Jack, the country professional man from our introduction? An environmental factor, wheat dust in the air, sparked off his allergic encephalitis. But it could only do so because the family's genetically transmitted grain allergies had made Jack vulnerable (other people live in the area with no problems at all).

So, it's not always a clear-cut case of environment on the one hand or genetics on the other. The best course, I believe, is to fill your family tree with all the evidence you can, and let your doctor determine causes on the basis of the total picture.

The kind of environmental information that's worth mentioning includes birthplaces (city or country, inland or coastal areas, which in earlier days influenced people's diets) and jobs (if granddad worked in an asbestos mine, that would explain his lung trouble and reassure you that it's not genetic).

Also worth mentioning, of course, are specific factors such as residence in soil-deficient areas or near a plant spewing out noxious wastes into the ground, water or air. And note any close association with animals, either on a farm or as household pets, as this can help to pinpoint

allergies and other links between animals and disease –
important both for diagnosis and research.

Valuable, too, is epidemiological information that
touches on personal habits. Alcoholism can sometimes be
a manifestation of grain or yeast allergies, or a zinc deficiency. Vegetarianism is worth putting in for the reasons
outlined earlier. The inclusion of cigarette smoking, drug
abuse, coffee abuse, analgesic addiction and extensive
medication can help to exclude genetic causes for illnesses as well as suggest or confirm connections between
such practices and various diseases.

In some cases, the very craving for things like coffee
and certain drugs can be another tip of a family's
malabsorption, allergic or metabolic-deficiency iceberg.

RICH MAN, POOR MAN, BEGGAR MAN OR THIEF?

What of the final category of epidemiological information – the one about people's achievements in life? What
benefit is it to know whether an ancestor was a head of
state, a convicted bank robber or a humble clerk?

Such information is, I must admit, of interest value
only. And yet, that kind of value is not to be sneezed at.
We all need a sense of identity – and if you know what
sort of people have gone before you in the family line,
that sense of identity becomes a lot stronger.

It doesn't really matter if they were famous or notorious, successes or failures, good or bad. What does matter
is that they emerge as real flesh-and-blood people – so
that you see yourself as part of a unique and special group
that stretches back through time and space. Your family.

Perhaps you've a heritage to live up to. Or humble
origins to spur you on to greater things. Either way, your
family tree will tell you who you are, where you've come
from, and where you're going – healthwise at least – in,
the future.

More help with the epidemiological section of your
family tree will be found in Appendix E.

THE INFORMATION: WHERE DO YOU GET IT?

There's one vital question left. Where do you get all the information to put on your family tree? Not from weathered tombstones of family Bibles or old parish records in England. Those sources are invaluable if you're compiling a family tree that stretches back for centuries: but our purpose, of course, is rather different.

We're compiling a family tree in the interests of your family's health.

True, you need to include as many people as you can unearth. And true, the farther back you can go the better. But for a medically valuable family tree, it's absolutely vital to include good, solid, relevant medical information – the kind of information that I've outlined in this chapter.

In other words, it's not much use going back six generations if your medical information cuts out with your parents. So, where do you go to get that information?

You go to your relatives, including, and especially, the oldest surviving ones that you have.

You can, of course, ring them up, write to them or drop in for afternoon tea. But there's another way that I've found to be not only simple, fast and highly effective, but great fun, too . . . hold a family tree party.

Send the invitations far and wide – uncles, aunts, cousins, second cousins, parents, grandparents, great-aunts and great-uncles – as many relatives as you can reasonably trace and invite. You'll find that most of them will jump at the chance of a genuine family reunion: it's something that everybody talks about, but hardly anyone does.

If possible, explain the purpose of the gathering when you issue invitations, so that people can think about the subject beforehand.

When everyone comes together, you'll naturally spend quite a while catching up – lots of people there won't have seen each other for years – and, generally, having a great time.

But, eventually, you'll get around to the purpose of the gathering. And the first thing to do is to put down the foundation of your family tree – the people themselves.

You'll probably know who your immediate forebears were, for a couple of generations anyway. But most people know surprisingly little about their grandparents' families, and even less about their great-grandparents. That's where the older relatives can fill you in, while the cousins can help you to expand the tree sideways.

Once the skeleton is complete, you can start adding the flesh – the relevant medical information and clues. Ask everyone to recall their memories about past generations – illnesses, causes of death, symptoms, signs, congenital conditions, phenotypes, environmental snippets – not forgetting, of course, the same information about themselves.

Write it all down carefully. Or tape-record it, if that's easier, and transcribe it later. Perhaps the best idea is to give everyone a questionnaire (see Appendix F at the back of the book for a sample) and use that as the basis of information gathering and discussion.

You'll be surprised at the amount of data that emerges. In all probability, there'll be enough for you to cover all the categories of information outlined in this chapter. And if you can produce a family tree as detailed as that, you'll have done something really significant, not only for your family's health, but perhaps for medical research, too.

However, even if your family tree finishes up with only the basics on it – known medical conditions, symptoms and signs – you'll still have something very worthwhile. Something that will give your doctor a flying start in diagnosing, treating and preventing your family's illnesses. Something that could make the difference in your family between health and disease, hope and despair – even life and death.

Now and for generations to come.

❖7❖

From Colds to Cancer: New Protection From Your Family Tree

Let's assume that the task is completed. You've held your family tree party. You have a pile of information. You've sifted it, digested it and finally written it down on a series of detailed, categorized family trees.

Now – what does it all mean? What are the things to look for: the things that can not only throw new light on your family's current medical problems, but warn you of trouble ahead, years before it strikes? They are, of course, many and varied. Several books would be necessary to look at them all in detail. So, to keep the next four chapters to a reasonable length, we'll look at the main ones – those that give definite warnings of the illnesses that loom as the biggest bogeymen in most people's minds.

Namely, cancer, heart disease, strokes, dementias and psychoses. We'll also discuss what you can do about them.

But, before we start, let's make two short digressions, beginning with a brief look at some illnesses that are a lot less scary than those listed above, but are even more widespread.

THE NUISANCE AILMENTS

In these next chapters, we'll see more evidence that your family tree is your staunchest ally in the fight against major illnesses. But it's important to realize that it can be just as valuable if your family is plagued by lesser ailments.

You know the things I mean – illnesses that often don't need the doctor, but have the knack of upsetting

123

routines and spoiling arrangements as well as making you and your family feel thoroughly miserable. Does there, for instance, always seem to be someone in your family with a cold? Do you all get flu every winter? Do the children pick up every childhood viral ailment that's going around – mumps, measles, chickenpox, German measles, 24-hour fevers?

Do you find your colds and sore throats tend to linger longer than average? And is there a constant stream of sniffles, swollen glands, middle-ear infections, coughs and bronchitis passing through your home?

Yes? Then one of two things is probably happening.

If the problems are things like recurring sniffles, wheezy coughs and minor skin disorders, allergies are the most likely cause. And if your family tree contains people with known allergic conditions such as asthma, hay fever, eczema or hives, the likelihood is a near certainty.

Just ask your doctor to refer you and your sniffles, coughs and itches to an allergist, and you're well on the way to relief.

It's a little more complicated when you're bothered by actual infections rather than allergic reactions. Then you start by asking the question: *why* is your family succumbing to regular viral and bacterial infections? What's happening to suppress your immune systems and make you easy prey for every passing bug?

The most likely reason is food allergies – and the vitamin/mineral deficiencies that flow from them. We touched, you'll recall, on immune-system suppression in Chapter 3. There we saw that it opens the door to many unpleasant diseases, right up to and including cancer. But it does the same for many minor ones, too, plus lots of in-between ones like glandular fever and hepatitis.

That's not hard to understand. A suppressed immune system simply means that your body can't fight viruses and bacteria as effectively as it should. Consequently, you pick up infections more easily and find it harder to get rid of them.

So, if your family is bothered by a seemingly nonstop series of minor and mildly serious infections, don't just suffer in silence. You'll find it very worthwhile to have your food allergies and vitamin-mineral levels checked. That's especially true if your family tree contains the classic food allergy indications (particularly to grains) that we've listed several times – prematurely gray hair, arthritis, bowel cancer, pernicious anemia, thyroid trouble, celiac disease, SLE, early baldness, chronic indigestion and frequent diarrhea.

By identifying your allergies, avoiding the guilty foods and taking the appropriate vitamins and minerals, you'll be surprised at the dramatic drop in your family's infection rate. You'll also drastically reduce the possibility of much more serious illnesses later on.

Which brings me back to the serious illnesses. And I'll lead into them by making our second brief digression.

A WORD OF REASSURANCE

The next four chapters will introduce you to a lot of conditions that, when appearing in a family tree, can be warnings of serious illnesses to come.

Before we look at them in detail, I want to add a word of reassurance. If some ominous things do feature in your family tree, please don't panic. Please don't assume that you're absolutely locked in to getting the foreshadowed disease. That's not what the warnings mean at all.

What they do mean is that your chances of getting that disease are somewhat higher than the community average. If there are only one or two warning signs in your family tree, your chances may only be very little above the normal. If there are lots of signs, then your chances are correspondingly higher.

Even so, please don't rush out tomorrow and start arranging your funeral. Your likelihood of avoiding the disease is still greater than your chance of getting it. And the warning that comes from your family tree will be a vital factor in keeping you healthy. Even when you're most at risk for one of those unpleasant illnesses, your doctor can almost always take positive action to protect you – once he or she is alerted to the risk.

With those comforting words ringing in our ears, let's devote this chapter to what is possibly the most feared illness of all.

Cancer.

Probably more books have been written on cancer than on any other illness. And probably no other illness is being so exhaustively studied, probed, theorized about and researched, all over the world. So, can anything new about cancer possibly be said in a book about family trees? The answer is definitely "yes," for two important reasons.

First, your family tree can, in very many cases, give you clear warning that you are a cancer risk. The significance of that hardly needs stressing, because an early warning of cancer usually leads to its early detection, which gives you the best possible chance of a total cure.

Second, your family tree can quite often, I believe, give vital clues to the biggest question of all: Why is cancer running through your family? Anything that can start to answer that question has, I'm sure you'll agree, enormous implications for cancer research and treatment. I'll back my claims with some hard evidence in Chapter 7.

Meanwhile, let's look at the conditions in your family tree that can indicate a raised cancer risk in you and your children.

CANCER-PRONE FAMILIES

The first condition is simply a family history of cancer. Despite what some people may tell you, cancer is not evenly distributed throughout the population. Some families have a great deal more of it than others – a growing body of evidence underlines that disturbing fact.

One American study looked at 4270 families on a random basis. Almost 3500 cases of cancer had occurred in those families; but they had occurred in only 2280 of them, or just 53.4 percent. No less than 46.6 percent of the families studied had any evidence of cancer at all.

In another American study, a mobile cancer detection unit in Nebraska, USA, screened 4515 people. Through a questionnaire and interviews, details were also obtained of any cases of cancer that had occurred in their close relatives. It was found that 9.84 percent of the people with one case of cancer in their family also had cancer themselves. The figure rose to 16.32 percent when two cases of cancer were in the immediate family, and to no less than 22.04 percent when the family had three or more cancer sufferers.

In both studies, the relationship between cancer in the family and an increased risk of getting it is plain to see.

The obvious question is, of course, why? Why are some families relatively prone to cancer, while others are much more resistant to it?

The evidence suggests that, if your family has a history of cancer, one of two things is happening. Either there is in your family some kind of hereditary cancer (the existence of which is now generally recognized), or some secondary hereditary factor is actually causing the cancer in your ranks. Many examples of cancer-prone families have now been discovered and written about, around the world. In the last few years, I've seen some spectacular ones myself, including one in which cancer struck twelve out of twelve sisters. We'll meet some of them in Chapter 11, including a family with eight cancer cases in two generations.

We'll also see just what else was running in those families – what was, I firmly believe, causing the cancers.

If there does happen to be cancer in your family tree, two more questions come immediately to mind. Can you tell whether the cancer itself is hereditary, or the secondary result of some other hereditary illness or condition? And does it matter, anyway?

To answer the second question first – yes, it matters very much indeed. If the cancer itself is hereditary, then about all you can do is be aware of the risk and have regular checkups.

But, if it's the secondary result of some other hereditary problem, that's a different story. You needn't just sit around waiting for the cancer to get you. You can take the offensive. Besides having regular checkups, you can take positive action to correct the problem, heading off the cancer before it happens.

There are, of course, plenty of cancers that just appear spontaneously in people who have no reason to expect them. However, a growing body of evidence does suggest that many cancers, perhaps even a majority, are either hereditary or the secondary result of hereditary problems.

With the help of your family tree, most of the hereditary ones can be predicted. And, as I've just indicated, many of those caused by hereditary problems can be prevented.

The first step is to decide which kind you're up against.

HEREDITARY CANCERS (AUTOSOMAL DOMINANT)

If your doctor is in touch with the latest discoveries about the genetics of cancer, he or she will be able to tell you if your family's cancers are hereditary. Many types of cancer are now known to be in this category. Their modes of transmission are pretty well understood, too. So your doctor will first look at the *kinds* of cancer in your family tree – and then at the *pattern* of their appearance in your family tree.

Say, for example, that retinoblastomas (tumors of the eye) are present. These are known to be hereditary in an autosomal dominant fashion. If there's just one case, it could be a spontaneous thing. But, if there are several cases, and they form an autosomal dominant pattern, you can be sure they are not spontaneous, but hereditary.

A glance at your family tree then shows you who has a 50 percent chance of getting them, and who should dodge them completely.

Many other autosomal dominant forms of cancer have now been recognized. They include at least four types of bowel cancer, including the Peutz-Jegher Syndrome – bowel cancer in association with brown patches on the lips and fingers. Also on the list are some thyroid cancers (especially one known as Sipple's Syndrome), melanomas of the skin or eye (some studies indicate that one in twelve melanomas may be hereditary), certain cancers of the adrenal gland and esophagus (the food tube from mouth to stomach) and carotid-body tumors.

The last-named are cancers of the carotid body, a nerve structure that regulates such basic body functions as breathing. And, a happy little thought I'll add in passing, if you do have a carotid-body tumor, you have an increased risk of getting an autosomal dominant cancer elsewhere in the body as well.

One particularly dangerous form of breast cancer is now thought to be autosomal dominant, too. It appears early, before the age of thirty, and usually in both breasts. So strong is the evidence for its autosomal dominant transmission that some American doctors are now studying family trees, identifying girls at risk, and carrying out preventative surgery – removing breast tissue and replacing it with a substitute – well before cancer symptoms have a chance to appear.

But it's not only this particular kind of breast cancer that may be hereditary. In fact, there's growing evidence that most breast cancers have some sort of genetic factors associated with them. The precise mode of transmission is not clear, but it's frequently been observed that close female relatives of breast-cancer victims have a greatly increased risk of getting it themselves. Some authorities put the risk as high as three times the normal level.

The male members of the family have no cause to sigh with relief, either. Several American studies have shown that all relatives, male and female, of breast-cancer sufferers run a much higher-than-normal risk of developing cancer in other parts of the body. The studies indicate

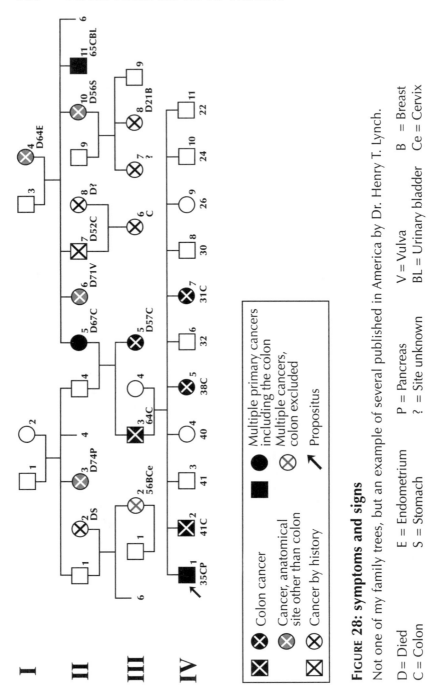

FIGURE 28: symptoms and signs

Not one of my family trees, but an example of several published in America by Dr. Henry T. Lynch.

D= Died	E = Endometrium	P = Pancreas	V = Vulva	B = Breast
C = Colon	S = Stomach	? = Site unknown	BL = Urinary bladder	Ce = Cervix

that, while almost any organ can be affected, cancers of the gastrointestinal tract, the ovaries, the prostate, the endometrium (the interior lining of the womb) and a combination of soft-tissue sarcomas, leukemia and brain tumors are particularly associated with breast cancer.

In other words, if breast cancer is running in your family, you need to be very much on your guard against other forms of cancer, too – especially those listed above.

What this appears to indicate is very significant indeed. Until fairly recently, it had been generally thought that hereditary cancers were *site-specific* – that is, they always appeared in the same organ, like retinoblastomas.

Now it seems that a tendency to get cancer in general, and not just a specific cancer, may be inherited. How this happens is not yet clear, but any doubts about the fact itself are rapidly being dispelled by more and more case histories.

Some researchers think the mechanisms may be partly genetic and partly environmental. They feel that some families may have a genetic factor that makes them particularly vulnerable to cancer-causing environmental agents – such as chemicals, viruses or cigarette smoke. Research into this possibility is continuing now in America.

THE CANCER FAMILY SYNDROME

The ultimate example of hereditary cancer rears its head in a phenomenon, which a top American authority calls the *cancer family syndrome*.

To gain membership in this fairly exclusive club, a family needs several unenviable qualifications. It must have an increased frequency of all cancers, especially in the colon and endometrium. About 20 percent or more of its cancer-victim members must have more than one primary cancer. The cancers must begin earlier in life than they normally do. And they must form an autosomal dominant pattern. American researchers have published details of many examples of the cancer family syndrome.

One family, known as "Family G," has been tracked continuously since 1895 and still shows no signs of losing its cancer-proneness.

Figure 28 (something of a milestone – it's the first family tree in the book that isn't one of mine) shows a typical example of the cancer family syndrome. It's one of several published by Dr. Henry T. Lynch, America's leading authority on cancer genetics.

Notice the number of cancer cases in just four generations, the early ages of onset, the multiple cancers in three out of eight people and the autosomal dominant pattern of transmission.

In families like this, close relatives of anyone with cancer have at least a 50 percent chance of developing cancer themselves. And here's the other interesting point; when the extended family (aunts, uncles, cousins, etc.) is added in, you invariably see the cancer following some branches of the family but not others – even when all share virtually the same environment.

That's another powerful pointer to the genetic origins of the cancer family syndrome.

So far, with the possible exception of ordinary breast cancer and the cancers associated with it, the hereditary cancers we've been examining are all autosomal dominant. Consequently, if they occur in that pattern in your family tree, you can safely assume that they are not chance happenings.

You can also see who has a 50 percent chance of becoming a victim, and who is probably not in the firing line.

I can't overemphasize the importance of that. It gives you the opportunity of early detection and an excellent chance of a total cure. Which, quite simply, is the difference between life and death – a difference made possible, in such a case, by your family tree.

AUTOSOMAL RECESSIVE CANCERS

Besides the autosomal dominant cancers – of which we have only looked at a few – there are some that seem to be autosomal recessive. These include neuroblastomas (cancers of the adrenal gland), Wilm's tumor (a form of kidney cancer), xeroderma pigmentosum (a rare but deadly kind of skin cancer) and some brain tumors.

Being autosomal recessive, they don't appear as inevitably as the autosomal dominant ones. In fact, they don't appear at all unless both parents carry matching recessive genes for them. But when that does happen, 25 percent of the couple's children, on the average, will be affected.

So, if you see any of those cancers heading toward you from both sides of your family, protect yourself with regular examinations – and catch and dispatch the cancer before it has time to cause trouble.

X-LINKED CANCERS

There are also some hereditary cancers that are X-linked or, perhaps more accurately, stem from a predisposition that is inherited in an X-linked way.

Chief among these are what are called the lympho-proliferative disorders, which include some bowel cancer, some brain tumors, certain varieties of leukemia, and some cases of Hodgkin's disease and lymphoma – the latter two being cancers of the lymph system.

The same process of deduction that we applied to the autosomal cancers holds good for the X-linked ones. If a cancer known to be X-linked is in fact occurring in that pattern in your family, you can assume that it's hereditary, and predict its future appearances accordingly.

From personal observation, I've come to suspect that a lot more cancers than those listed above have an X-linked genetic basis. I've noticed, for instance, that gastric cancer follows red-green color blindness in some families. I've also noticed, in other families, that cancer often goes along with manic-depressive illness.

Both those conditions are certainly X-linked. Their close association with cancer in many families is evidence, I believe, that in those cases, both they and the cancer spring from a common X-linked genetic factor. If so, anyone with color blindness or manic-depressive illness in such families has a very high risk of getting cancer too.

Because I've seen those and similar associations so often, I can't help feeling that X-linkage will prove to be a much more important factor in hereditary cancer than is currently realized. In fact, I have a theory: Namely, that when there's a great deal of nonautosomal cancer in a family, it will almost always be in an X-linked pattern.

I base that theory on my studies of several cancer-prone families, but more case histories are needed before I can assert it as a fact.

If I'm right, it means that nonautosomal familial cancer is either an X-linked phenomenon or (more probably) is caused by one or more X-linked hereditary factors. It also means that familial cancer can be predicted and prevented with much more certainty than is now believed to be the case. So, if there's a lot of nonautosomal cancer in your family, plot it on your family tree and see if it's X-linked. If it is, you'll help to prove my theory – and, more importantly, you'll see right away who's next in line.

PRECANCERS: HEREDITARY WARNINGS

As well as the hereditary cancers themselves, there are many conditions known as *precancers* that are also hereditary. These are conditions that positively shout a warning of cancer, whether they appear in you personally or in other members of your family.

Some experts believe that precancerous conditions are a direct cause of cancer. Others maintain that they and the cancer both spring from some common genetic factor. At this stage of medical knowledge, the question is unresolved. What is certain is this: A family tree full of precancerous conditions is as ominous as a family tree full of cancer itself.

Hereditary precancerous conditions come in autosomal dominant, autosomal recessive and X-linked varieties. So if they occur in your family tree, you can predict where they're likely to show up next. And when you do, treat them with the utmost seriousness: Anyone with one of these conditions has an above-average chance of getting cancer too.

We won't attempt to list all the known hereditary precancerous conditions, as over 160 have now been identified. We'll take a moment, though, to look at some of the more important examples.

AUTOSOMAL DOMINANT PRECANCERS

Among the autosomal dominant ones is von Recklinghausen's Syndrome. You'll recall that its outward manifestations are lumps and nodules all over the face and body, and that people who have it are at real risk for cancers of the brain and spinal cord.

Also autosomal dominant and worthy of note are three pre-cancerous conditions called exostosis, multiple intestinal polyposis, and (would you believe) keratosis palmaris et plantaris.

I'm probably safe in assuming that all three are new to you. So, in plain English, exostosis is the presence of bony spurs on the heels, hands, fingers or elsewhere. Multiple intestinal polyposis is numerous tiny polyps all over the interior walls of the intestine. And the last-named fugitive from a high school Latin class is a thickening of the skin on the palms of the hand and the soles of the feet.

The first two are closely linked with bowel cancer. In fact, people with multiple intestinal polyposis almost always get bowel cancer before they're fifty. And for some reason, people with keratosis palmeris et plantaris run a greatly increased risk of cancer of the esophagus.

What's more, if a direct forebear had any of these conditions, and if you're in the firing line, you have an increased risk of getting the cancer with which it's linked – even if you don't have the condition yourself.

AUTOSOMAL RECESSIVE PRECANCERS

As you digest that cheerful thought, let's take a quick look at some autosomal recessive precancers. They include albinism, and at least you know what that is. Others you'd be markedly less familiar with include Werner's Syndrome, Bloom's Syndrome, Fanconi's aplastic anemia and ataxia telangiectasia. The last two are hereditary anemias characterized by low white blood cell and platelet counts. Fanconi's is also accompanied by malformations of the heart, kidneys, hands and feet. Both carry with them a high risk for leukemia.

Bloom's Syndrome is a combination of low birth weight, sensitivity to sunlight and a tendency toward chromosomal breakdown and mutation. Here, again, leukemia is the undesirable fellow traveler. Werner's Syndrome is a kind of premature aging. It involves early hardening of the arteries, diabetes, premature graying, thickening of the skin on hands and feet, cataracts and calcifications under the skin. A strong link with gastrointestinal cancer makes that charming picture complete.

Albinism, of course, is a total lack of melanin pigment in the skin. Not surprisingly, skin cancer is its ever-present accomplice; although, in this case, probably as a direct result of the condition itself, rather than as a linked manifestation of a common genetic factor.

X-LINKED PRECANCERS

So far, only a few X-linked precancerous conditions have been identified. Two of these are the X-linked dominant Bruton's agammaglobulinemia (try saying that three times quickly) and the X-linked recessive Wiskott-Aldrich Syndrome.

Bruton's tongue twister is basically the absence of a certain type of white blood cell. This leads to the lack of an antibody group that guards against bacterial infection. As a result, sufferers are very prone to bacterial infections, plus such symptoms as rheumatoid arthritis.

Until the coming of antibiotics, they usually died at an early age. Now they mostly survive into adulthood – only to find that bowel cancers and lymphomas attack them at a considerably higher-than-average rate.

Survival into adulthood is still uncertain for people with the Wiskott-Aldrich Syndrome. The symptoms here are lots of infections and bowel disorders, coupled with eczema and low blood platelet counts. Both in childhood and adulthood, the outlook is bleak, because those who survive the syndrome itself face a high incidence of leukemia.

Neither the autosomal recessive nor the X-linked precancerous conditions appear in family trees as often as the autosomal dominant ones – the recessives because of their recessive nature, and the X-linked because they are so often fatal in childhood. But their significance is the same: whether or not you have it yourself, if one does bob up in your family tree and you're in the genetic line for it, your changes of getting its associated cancer are higher than normal.

However, there's one point I'd like to emphasize again. If you do have a family history of cancer or precancerous conditions, and your family tree shows you're at risk, it doesn't mean that you'll automatically get cancer. The chances are that you won't. But, if you know you're at risk, just have regular examinations – then, if cancer does develop, it will be detected early and almost certainly cured.

CANCERS CAUSED BY HEREDITARY CONDITIONS

Suppose on the other hand, that you're threatened by the second kind of predictable cancer – the kind that is actually caused by some other hereditary problem or condition. In that case, you can take much more positive action than simply having regular checkups and crossing your fingers.

I've seen several hundred families that fall into this second category. They are distinguished by an unusually high incidence of cancer – but not always the cancers that are known to be hereditary. The interesting thing is this: In almost every instance, there is something else also running through those families. Something else that we have met on several occasions before in this book. Something else that is definitely hereditary, and is, I am convinced, actually causing those above-average rates of cancer.

That something else is our old foe, autoimmune disease, in its various manifestations.

In some families it's there as pernicious anemia; in others, as celiac disease; in still others, as connective tissue disorders such as SLE and related illnesses like Sjogren's Syndrome, scleroderma and dermatomyositis.

Very often, it surfaces as a whole cluster of such things. I've seen family after family with both pernicious anemia and celiac disease, usually with thyroid disorders, arthritis and diabetes thrown in, too. I've seen lots of others in which that same cluster is accompanied by SLE. And in a very high percentage of all of them, the number of cancer cases is way above average.

Autoimmune disease is not a widely recognized thing among nonmedical people. You don't find people discussing it at parties, the way they discuss better-known afflictions. And yet, as you've probably gathered by now, I think it's one of the most important – and most overlooked – causes of serious illness that we've yet discovered.

In earlier chapters, we saw how it leads to a wide range of psychiatric symptoms and causes tissue damage in various parts of the body. Now we're considering its links with cancer. And in a while, we'll study its implications in things like presenile dementia and thromboses.

This all adds up to a pretty impressive criminal record. In fact, about the only good thing about autoimmune disease is that it shows up so plainly in a family tree. As a result, it telegraphs its punches so clearly that you can usually duck before they connect.

THE LINK BETWEEN AUTOIMMUNE DISEASE AND CANCER

How, exactly, does autoimmune disease lead to an increased risk for cancer? I believe the mechanism works something like this.

Autoimmune disease goes hand-in-hand with food allergies. Indeed, as we saw in a previous chapter, there's good evidence that food allergies actually cause it. Be that as it may, it's certainly my experience that you rarely find autoimmune disease in a family without accompanying food allergies. Now, as we've also seen, food allergies prevent the body from properly absorbing most essential vitamins and minerals. The deficiencies that result lead to all kinds of health problems – and perhaps the most serious of these is an impaired, or suppressed, immune system.

What are the signs of immune system suppression? A family tree with an unusually high incidence and frequency of viral infections: severe colds, hepatitis, flu and glandular fever. If this is happening in your family, be on your guard. An impaired immune system lays out the welcome mat for a whole host of unpleasant diseases. One of which, according to recent research, is cancer.

So the link is clear at that level. The presence of autoimmune disease suggests food allergies; the presence of food allergies leads to a damaged immune system; and a damaged immune system seriously predisposes you for cancer.

It takes many years for cancer to develop from the immune-system-suppressing activities of food allergies. But in some families, I believe the process gets under way at a very early age indeed: the tender age, in fact, of six or seven months or more *before* birth.

IS CANCER A CONGENITAL DISORDER?

Here, admittedly, I am venturing somewhat into the realm of theory – but there is strong and growing evidence for my beliefs, which began with the following solidly proven facts. They may seem unrelated at first, but their significance will soon be clear.

Fact number one: During pregnancy, the placenta releases hormones that play a vital part in the formation (or *differentiation*, to use the technical term) of fetal tissues. Interestingly enough, the fetus's own adrenal cortex plays a major role in this operation. It secretes a substance called DHEAS, (dehydroepiandrosterone) which stimulates the placenta into releasing estrogens – specialized hormones that are also very important for fetal tissue development. To work normally, the whole process needs an adequate supply of vitamins and minerals from the mother.

Fact number two: When someone is highly allergic to grains, milk, eggs, beef and yeast, the substances that actually do the damage are what are known as *subfractions* – the components of the grains, milk, eggs, beef and yeast. Among these are gluten, α-gliadin, α-casein, secalin and hordein in grains and yeast, and (take a deep breath) α-lactalbumins and β-lactoglobulins in milk, eggs and beef.

Fact number three: when people have grain, milk, egg, beef and yeast allergies, they do not absorb vitamins and minerals properly from their food. Consequently, as we have seen several times, they are very often severely deficient in essential vitamins and minerals.

Now for the theory. I believe that, when women with such allergies are pregnant, their vitamin-mineral deficiencies do two sinister things. They prevent the placenta from releasing the normal amount of hormones. And they reduce the supply of vitamins and minerals that reaches the fetus.

This second action not only lowers the fetus's vitamin-mineral levels, but also means that less DHEAS is being released from its adrenal cortex, which interferes with the supply of estrogens from the placenta.

That all adds up to an abnormal balance within the fetus of hormones, vitamins and minerals. Nor is that the whole story. I think that further significant damage is caused by the toxic subfractions of the foods to which the mother is allergic – and which are toxic to the fetus too, if the sensitivity to them has been passed on to it genetically.

These subfractions, I believe, cross the placenta and can actually take the place of some of the hormones that are, for the reasons outlined above, in short supply. In other words, the toxic subfractions may actually have a hormonelike action on the fetus.

The net result of the faulty hormone-vitamin-mineral balance, plus the presence and hormonelike action of the toxic food fractions, is that some of the fetus's tissues are laid down abnormally. Formed before the immune system has matured, these tissues have a special metabolism that makes them different from normal cells. They are, in fact, *premalignant*. That is, they are especially likely to go wild and proliferate in later life, if exposed again to the toxic food fractions and the faulty hormone-vitamin-mineral environment that originally helped to form them.

What makes that proliferation happen, in my view? Please follow me carefully while I seek to explain. Throughout our body, some of our cells have what are called *receptors* for various hormones, proteins, enzymes and other substances. Through these, the cell receives what it needs for normal growth and division. Each receptor is specially designed to receive one particular kind or hormone, protein or enzyme.

The cells in the *premalignant* tissue, however, also have receptors for the toxic food fractions that helped to form them because those fractions, you'll remember, took the place of some normal hormones in the womb.

So, sooner or later, the person with food allergies will have those toxic food fractions crossing into their bloodstream and hovering around the cells with receptors for them. At the same time, the fractions will suppress the person's immune system, and upset his or her overall balance of hormones, vitamins and minerals.

When that happens, the faulty environment that caused the abnormal tissue to be formed has recurred.

Then, I believe, the cells in that tissue take in the toxic food fractions, just as they did in the womb. And, just as they did in the womb, the fractions stimulate the cells to proliferate and reproduce – only this time there are no in-utero growth-regulating hormones to keep the process in check. So the cells proliferate wildly and uncontrollably. And when they do so, cancer has begun.

In other words, I believe that cancer in many families is really a congenital disorder – begun by the effect of food allergies on the developing fetus, and exploding into life when the faulty prebirth environment recurs.

According to my theory, then, such cancers are actually mimicking the rapid proliferation of fetal tissues. Or, if you like, they are really abnormal fetal tissues starting to proliferate all over again. I think it's significant for my theory that many cancer cells do, in fact, release fetal proteins, which are normally seen only in unborn babies.

However, as I said, further research is needed to establish the total accuracy of this picture. But it would certainly explain why cancer occurs with frightening frequency in autoimmune-disease/food-allergy families. On the basis of my experience, I believe firmly that every cancer patient should be tested for the presence of antibodies to the subfractions of grains, milk, eggs, beef and yeast . . . especially if there are food allergies in his or her family tree.

If those tests are carried out, there are real and exciting possibilities for a total cure. I've seen it happen several times, as the case histories in Chapter 11 will demonstrate.

It's pretty logical, after all. If food allergies are running in the family, they are very likely to be present in the cancer patient. If so, they will be hard at work on four tasks: creating telltale autoantibodies; suppressing the immune system; reestablishing the faulty prebirth environment that helped form premalignant tissue; and (I believe) acting as growth factors for the cancer cells, if those cells have receptors for them.

Consequently, continues my theory, if the allergies and toxic food fractions are identified and the patient totally avoids the offending foods, all four processes will be reversed. The production of autoantibodies will be halted. The suppression of the immune system will stop. When appropriate vitamin-mineral supplements are added, the faulty hormone-vitamin-mineral environment will disappear. And, most important of all, the toxic food fractions that are essential to the cancer cells' growth and proliferation will be removed.

When those things happen, the body's natural defenses against cancer will be back in business. Cancer treatments will suddenly be more effective – in many cases, the cancer will actually stop growing, shrink or go away. And, in some, a complete and permanent cure will be achieved.

What's more, if this theory is correct, it could lead to the development of new anticancer drugs that would actually be attracted to the cancer cells' receptors, just like the toxic food fractions are; but instead of nourishing the cells, the drugs would destroy them.

Another possibility is to inject the patient with minute amounts of toxic fractions that have been *tagged* with a radioactive tracer. These would then travel to the cancer site and, via a full-body scintillograph, tell the doctor just where the cancer was, and its size and severity.

Controversial? Yes. Likely to be dismissed out of hand by many doctors? Undoubtedly. But it's a theory firmly based on what I have seen. And there are too many case histories building up for it to be lightly set aside. After you read Chapter 11, I think you'll agree.

Meanwhile, I'll take the theory one logical step further.

HEREDITARY CANCER – OR HEREDITARY CAUSE?

A few pages back, I said there are two kinds of cancers that run in families – type one, that is directly hereditary, and type two, that is the secondary result of other hereditary illnesses or conditions.

I'm now going to suggest that many of the type ones we discussed at length are really, in fact, type twos.

In other words, I believe that many cancers now generally classified as hereditary are actually the secondary results of the hereditary conditions – specifically, autoimmune disease and food allergies – but that few people have yet noticed the high incidence of such conditions in cancer-prone families.

I would love to know, for example, what else is running through those families we looked at previously – the ones with the cancer family syndrome. The researchers haven't looked at that aspect: they've just tracked and recorded the actual cancers.

So there's a giant new area for research. We know for sure that many cancers are hereditary. What we don't know is what percentage is caused by other hereditary conditions.

The difference is crucial. Those of the first kind can only be overcome by passive means: awareness of the risk, regular examinations and treatment when the cancer occurs. Those of the second kind can be attacked much more positively. Indeed, if the cause is identified, and positive action taken to eliminate it, the cancer can be prevented from occurring at all. Even if it has begun, removal of the factors that are causing or stimulating it will be a huge step toward a total cure.

Perhaps the most exciting thing about this new field of cancer research – this proof to determine whether a cancer is primarily or secondarily hereditary, a type one or type two – is that it's not confined to high-powered scientists with mind-boggling equipment in space-age laboratories. It can be carried out by ordinary people who have no medical or scientific training – because there's only one tool required for it.

The family tree.

As more and more people with cancer in their families compile detailed family trees, we will see more and more clearly the factors that accompany cancer in its murderous path. Of these, I am convinced that hereditary autoimmune disease will prove to be the most important.

Just imagine the implications if I'm right. Many, many cases of cancer will be predicted and prevented before they even begin. Many, many more will have their growth dramatically slowed or halted or be completely cured. Far fewer people will be born with premalignant tissue. Because of the prediction and prevention made possible by the family tree approach, there will be enormous savings in costs, as well as in lives and suffering.

What's more, all of this can happen on one of history's smallest research budgets – the cost of some paper and pencils, and the time and effort involved in getting the family together.

Don't get me wrong. I'm not saying that all hereditary cancers will turn out to be type twos. There is certainly a hard core of type ones – autosomal and X-linked. There is certainly an hereditary tendency to get cancer in general. And, of course, the family tree approach is a lifesaver in those instances, too, because it tells you who's at risk and needs to have the regular examinations that lead to early detection and an almost certain cure.

In addition, if enough family trees containing type-one cancers are compiled, they could help to reveal what is actually being inherited, and shed new light on how these cancers are being transmitted. That could well lead to breakthroughs in their prevention and treatment.

CANCER IN YOUR FAMILY? DO THIS NOW!

But meanwhile, I really want to emphasize this. If cancer appears frequently in your family, see if your family tree contains cases of known food allergies (especially to grains and milk), pernicious anemia, celiac disease, SLE or other connective tissue disorders, thyroid problems, arthritis, diabetes, premature graying or recurring viral infections. If it does, have yourself and your family tested without delay for food allergies and autoimmune disease.

Don't wait while the "experts" argue. Find out right away whether you and your loved ones have those conditions. Do so even if the cancer in your family appears to be a known hereditary type.

Should the tests prove positive, avoid the offending foods as if they were poison. Have the autoimmune disease treated promptly and thoroughly. If I'm wrong, you'll at least live a healthier and happier life. And if I'm right, you'll almost certainly avoid the cancer that has attacked other members of your family.

Right now, vast sums of money and the totally dedicated efforts of brilliant minds are being poured into cancer research. Wouldn't it be ironic if major breakthroughs in cancer prediction, prevention and treatment were made just by ordinary people compiling their family trees?

Yet, if enough ordinary people do so, I'm convinced that this will indeed be the case.

☆8☆

Fight Dementia with Your Family Tree

For all its spine-tingling associations, cancer isn't the only disease that people lie awake and worry about. Dementia, I find, is something else that really strikes fear into the relatives of people who develop it.

By *dementia*, I mean the symptoms of severe mental confusion, such as frequently accompany old age, appearing in people quite a bit younger than you would normally expect.

We all know, or have heard of, people in this category: those who aren't very old, but who forget their name and where they live and what day it is. Finally they have to be put into a home, both for their sake and that of their families. The relatives then look at themselves and start wondering, "Will the same thing happen to me?"

Perhaps you're in that situation. And wondering . . .

If you are, there's an excellent chance that your family tree will give you the answer. But even more importantly, if the answer is "yes, it could happen to you," your family tree will, in most cases, tell you how to make sure it doesn't.

Let's look (*Figure 29*) at a hypothetical family tree that shows the kind of pattern I've seen time and again in dementia families.

Two dementias in generation one. Things like prematurely graying hair, celiac disease, gastric cancer, depression and chronic lack of energy in generation two. Then hyperactivity, learning difficulties, behavioral problems and frequent viral infections among the children in generation three.

That might seem a pretty varied collection of ailments, but there's one common factor behind them all – grain

147

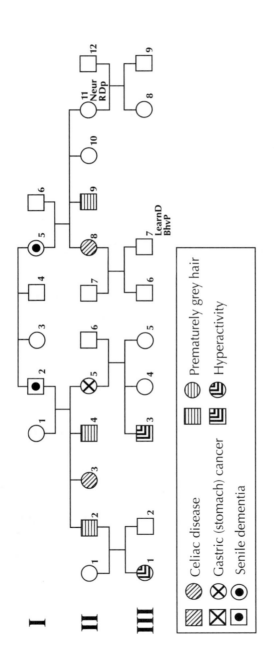

FIGURE 29: dementia

This hypothetical family tree shows the kind of pattern typically found in dementia families.

Bhv P	= Behavioral problems	Neur = Neurasthenia (chronic lack of energy)
Learn D	= Learning difficulties	R Dp = Recurring depression

allergies. Such a picture, in fact, is an absolutely classic grain allergy one. And, I stress again, it's precisely the picture that crops up over and over in dementia families. When you see it you can bet your boots that the allergy is hereditary, and is actually causing all these illnesses and conditions.

Including the dementias.

Now, I'm not saying that all dementias are caused by grain allergies. But there's no doubt whatsoever that grain allergies can cause them. So when you see dementias in a family that's loaded with grain-allergy manifestations, you don't have to be Sherlock Holmes to deduce the dementias' most likely cause.

Or to realize whom else in the family is at risk for them. Grain allergies don't always lead to dementias; when they do, it's because of something in that particular family's genetic makeup. This means that everyone else in the family with grain-allergy-induced problems needs to beware of dementia too.

The good news is the clear warnings offered by the family tree. As soon as you see a pattern like that, you know precisely what to do. You identify the offending grains with the appropriate allergy tests. The people affected avoid those grains like the plague, and have the associated vitamin-mineral deficiencies corrected.

In so doing, they should avoid the dementia too – as well as achieving a very significant improvement in their other health problems.

So, if there are dementias in your family, think first of grain allergies, and check your family tree for visible evidence of their presence.

INDICATIONS OF GRAIN ALLERGY

The signs of grain allergies include the things we've just seen in our hypothetical family tree: prematurely gray hair, celiac disease, gastric cancer, depression with chronic lack of energy, frequent infections, and hyperactivity and learning difficulties in children. They also include pernicious anemia, pellagra (low Vitamin B$_3$), SLE, thyroid disorders and diabetes.

When some or all of these appear in a dementia-plagued family, you're on pretty safe ground in assuming that the dementias are the result of grain allergies – or more specifically, of the savage deficiencies in Vitamins B$_3$, B$_{12}$, B$_1$ and folic acid (another B-group vitamin) and minerals such as zinc, magnesium and manganese, which the grain allergies cause.

That means, as I said a moment ago, that dementias in such families are almost totally avoidable – and many are reversible even once they've begun.

A good example is dementia caused by pellagra, a massive grain-allergy-induced Vitamin B$_3$ deficiency. Many doctors will tell you that pellagra is rare. On the contrary, I've found it to be surprisingly common. It's a condition that turns up with some regularity when you investigate a family with grain-allergy signs.

People with pellagra often have a telltale fissure down the middle of their tongues (looked at your tongue in the mirror lately?). They also tend to have chronic diarrhea and dermatitis as well as a high incidence of dementia – a syndrome sometimes rather irreverently called the "Three D's."

Yet, for all its nastiness, pellagra obediently fades away with large doses of Vitamin B$_3$. The dementias of which it warns can be avoided in almost every case. Even those already under way can usually be reversed, provided treatment begins within a year or two of their appearance.

DEMENTIAS WITH A DOUBLE CAUSE

Among the grain-allergy manifestations listed above, you'll note that I've included afflictions such as thyroid disorders, diabetes, pernicious anemia and SLE.

Am I thereby asserting that such things are always and only caused by grain allergies?

No, I'm not. But it's certainly true, in my experience, that all four conditions are more commonly seen in grain-allergy families – so much so, that their very appearance makes you wonder whether you've found another such family before a single allergy test is done. And when those conditions do appear in grain-allergy families, the chances of dementias occurring there too are considerably increased, for a twofold reason.

First, thyroid disorders, diabetes, pernicious anemia and SLE can themselves cause dementias. And second, as we've seen, grain allergies can too, by triggering off massive mineral and B-group vitamin deficiencies. Grain allergies, in fact, can even be the direct cause of central nervous system degeneration.

So, when one of the above conditions and grain allergies are a duo act, they tend to reinforce each other's dementia-causing properties – a reinforcement the family could well do without.

Consequently, if grain allergies are in your family tree, it's important to establish whether thyroid disorders, diabetes, pernicious anemia and SLE are in there with them.

However, that may not be quite as easy as it sounds.

We've noted on a number of occasions that thyroid disorders, pernicious anemia and SLE are all notorious for being misdiagnosed or missed altogether. Diabetes is less frequently overlooked these days, although it often was in the past. It's possible that these conditions may have occurred in your family, but have never been diagnosed by name. That makes it a little harder to put them in your family tree. Harder, but by no means impossible – if they have visited your family, they'll have left behind clear signs of their presence.

Take SLE, for instance. If there are grain allergies in your family, but no known cases of SLE, there may be or have been people with vague aches and pains, or who burnt easily in the sun, or who were losing their hair at an early age, or had migraine, arthritis, depressive illness or chronic lack of energy.

All those things can accompany SLE. So can recurring mouth ulcers, frequent infections (especially of the bladder and upper respiratory tract), butterfly rash on the face, hands that go cold and blue, minor strokes – and, of course, dementias.

On their own, none of those things automatically means SLE. But, if there's a fair sprinkling of them in your family tree, there's a very good chance that SLE has been or is there, too, unrecognized and undiagnosed. And if yours is also a grain-allergy family, that means dementias are a real possibility to be watched for and guarded against.

Or take thyroid disorders. Are there, or have there been, people in your family who are overweight and tend to be sluggish and depressed, with deep voices, high blood pressure and varicose veins? If so, you have good reason to suspect undiagnosed thyroid disorders – especially if any of those people also became demented, or if dementias have appeared elsewhere in your family.

Other possible pointers to thyroid trouble include symptoms and signs like poor memory, sallow complexion, coarse features, early deafness, heavy and painful periods in women, cold hands and carpal tunnel syndrome (pains in the wrist). Once again, the combination of those things and grain allergies in your family tree sound a definite dementia warning. In a moment, we'll discuss how you can effectively respond to it.

Meanwhile, let's consider diabetes. If that has cropped up recently in your family, it will almost certainly have been diagnosed as such, and you'll have no trouble putting it in the family tree.

However, if it occurred two or three generations ago, it may well have been missed. But you need to know about it if it did occur, to accurately assess your family's dementia risk.

So, if you know there are grain allergies in your family, your next move is to check your family tree for people with the following problems . . . cataracts, leg amputations, recurring boils, strokes, heart attacks, a "sweet tooth," sudden loss of weight or congenital abnormalities.

It's also worth noting mothers who had babies over 4.5 kg.

If only one or two of these appear, the case for diabetes would remain unproved. But if there are a number of them, and especially if the same people developed dementias, there's a high probability that diabetes has joined forces with grain allergies to plot your family's downfall – and to boost your chances of developing dementia.

However, the plot can be fairly easily thwarted, as we'll shortly see.

Lastly, there is pernicious anemia. Here's another elusive ailment that can smolder away for years and cause all sorts of problems, including dementias, without ever being firmly pinned down and diagnosed.

Fortunately, however, while it might avoid being identified by name, it can't avoid leaving its footsteps in the family tree. Suspect undiagnosed pernicious anemia if, in your grain-allergy-affected family, there are people with prematurely gray hair, chronic indigestion, frequent diarrhea, shiny red and sore tongues, anemia, broad foreheads or sallow complexions.

Another giveaway is an ancestor who, on doctor's orders, used to eat raw liver. This seemingly bizarre practice was actually an old treatment for pernicious anemia – and not a bad one, either.

But one of the nastiest things about pernicious anemia is that, while it can certainly cause dementias on its own, it's even more likely to do so when gastric cancer is also in the family.

People who have both are quite high dementia risks, especially if other dementia cases have already occurred in the family. Consequently, if your family has cases of gastric cancer and pernicious anemia – or a sampling of the symptoms and signs I've just listed – as well as grain allergies, dementias are something you need to keep in mind.

Before they blow your mind.

How to avoid grain-allergy-linked dementias

Now we come to the real point of the exercise: protecting you and your family from dementias caused by grain allergies, and from those caused by a combination of grain allergies and thyroid disorders, diabetes, pernicious anemia or SLE.

If grain allergies seem to be the sole culprits, the process is fairly simple – surprisingly simple, when you consider how devastating the allergies can be if left untreated.

As I said a few pages back, the first step is to use allergy tests to identify the offending grains. If you and your family are affected, you then avoid those grains as if they were poison (which, as far as you're concerned, they are). You also take the right vitamins and minerals to help repair any tissue damage that may already have been done.

Those steps should slash your risks for dementia almost to zero, and they will give any relatives with recent dementias a real chance of regaining their right minds.

The process is a little more involved when the grain-allergy threat is compounded by one of the other four hangers-on. But the pathway to prevention and frequent cures is still plain to see.

If thyroid disorders are complicating the grain-allergy picture, you add thyroxin to the above line of treatment. If it's diabetes, diet and/or insulin therapy is the additional step. If it's pernicious anemia, intramuscular injections of Vitamin B_{12} will probably be required. And if it's SLE, a course of cortisone may be needed, along with the total avoidance of milk and grains.

The point to be emphasized is this: The family tree approach can provide the vital diagnostic information needed to prevent or cure almost all dementia cases caused by grain allergies, pellagra, thyroid disorders, diabetes, pernicious anemia or SLE. Hundreds of thousands of people can be freed to live normal, independent, mentally alert lives, instead of being shoved into nursing homes. Just consider the relief of human misery that represents – and the savings in health care costs.

But, of course, not all dementias are caused by grain allergies and their associated illnesses. Can the family tree approach be of value when grain allergies don't seem to be to blame?

It certainly can – because there do appear to be genetic factors at work in at least some of the other dementias. And one of the worst of them is definitely known to be autosomal dominant.

HUNTINGTON'S CHOREA: A GENETIC TRAGEDY

This latter one, Huntington's chorea, is the devastating dementia that we touched on briefly in Chapter 2. As we saw then, the tragedy of Huntington's chorea is that it usually shows up in later life, well after people have had children, hence, after they have already passed on the gene for it to the next generation.

Equally tragic are the symptoms that the disease produces in its victims.

It often begins with an unusual or staggering gait – a symptom that sometimes sees the sufferer picked up by the police for drunkenness. Severe personality changes are also typical. Pleasant, mild people may become violent and aggressive, or deeply depressed and suicidal. They may exhibit symptoms very like those of paranoid schizophrenia. Then, they may develop uncontrollable body movements before plunging into a dark and hopeless dementia.

Not a pretty picture – but, as you can imagine, one that really stands out in a family tree.

If you're unlucky enough to have a Huntington's chorea in your family, it will almost certainly have been diagnosed as such, and you'll already know about it. But even if it hasn't been diagnosed, your family tree will quickly point to its presence. A family history of personality change leading to violent behavior, suicide or confinement to institutions, with the affected people linked together in an autosomal dominant pattern, would give you a virtually firm diagnosis.

The terrible thing, however, is this: The children of people with Huntington's chorea have one chance in two of developing the disease themselves because of its autosomal dominant transmission. And there's really nothing you can do to prevent it.

About the only possible action is to keep as fit and healthy as you can. There's some evidence that physical fitness may delay the condition's onset. But a delay is all it will achieve. It won't prevent the disease from developing if you've inherited the guilty gene.

The only ray of hope in the whole situation is that the disease can at least be stopped from going past the present generation. If one of your parents had Huntington's chorea, don't have children yourself. There's a 50 percent chance that your sacrifice will be in vain, and that you won't develop the disease after all. But on the other hand, if you do develop it, half your children probably would too – so the tragic cycle would go on.

On a happier note, if one of your grandparents had it, but your aged parent (that grandparent's offspring) didn't, then you're perfectly safe. Your parent escaped the faulty gene and, obviously, couldn't have passed it on to you.

In that case, be fruitful, multiply and enjoy your children.

OTHER GENETICALLY BASED DEMENTIAS

What about genetic factors in other forms of dementia? Recent studies point strongly to their existence, and underline the importance of the family tree in determining your degree of risk.

A well-compiled family tree will certainly tell you the first thing you need to know – the ages at which people in your family developed dementias. If they were over seventy, it seems that there is little genetic dementia risk to their close relatives.

On the other hand, if at least two people under sixty-five have become victims, the risk to others in the family is quite considerable. In fact, when someone becomes demented early, and had a parent who did as well, nearly half of his or her brothers and sisters will also develop dementia.

By now, you'll recognize that particular pattern as an autosomal dominant one – or apparently so. And such a pattern has been observed in several presenile dementias, including those known as Alzheimer's disease, Pick's disease, Creutzfeldt-Jakob disease, and kuru.

However, there are some intriguing twists to the way these conditions seem to be transmitted.

Twist number one: If you take certain viruslike particles from the brains of people with Alzheimer's disease or Creutzfeldt-Jakob disease, and inject them into animals, the unfortunate creatures will develop many of the disease's symptoms.

Twist number two: Creutzfeldt-Jakob disease was once transmitted to a patient who received a cornea transplant from the eye of a sufferer.

Twist number three: In parts of Papua, New Guinea, whole villages have been devastated by a strange dementialike disease called kuru. This appeared to have an autosomal dominant pattern of transmission, until it was found to be passed on via a local custom of honoring deceased relatives by eating their brains.

All of which seems to point to a viral agent at work in these kinds of dementia. But there's a catch to that as a total explanation, too.

The catch is simply this: The family trees of people with those dementias are just too close to an autosomal dominant pattern to be purely the result of viruses. That is, in these families, the typical picture is a presenile dementia sufferer with around 50 percent of his or her children also becoming demented. If slow-acting viruses were the sole cause, you would expect the disease to appear in more than just 50 percent of those at risk for it.

Some researchers believe that what we have here is a combination of a slow virus and a genetic susceptibility to it. In other words, there may indeed be a slow-acting virus for presenile dementias, and it could be transmitted from one generation to another in your family. But whether it affects you or not would depend on your personal genetic makeup.

From our point of view in this book, it doesn't really matter whether that theory is right, or if genetic transmission is the main factor involved. Either way, your family tree is invaluable in plotting the dementia's path through your family, and in telling you whether or not you or your children are likely to become victims.

And what if you are? Can anything be done to protect you from Alzheimer's disease and similar presenile dementias?

Unfortunately, in the light of current medical knowledge, it would appear not. But then, on the other hand . . .

The operative word in that gloomy forecast is "current." On the basis of several dozen family trees I have now seen, I think some very interesting discoveries are just around the corner. The fascinating thing in these family trees is the other conditions that consistently show up along with Alzheimer's disease. In particular, they include lymphomas (bowel cancers) and Down's Syndrome (mongolism).

Now, what is that telling us about those conditions? Is there a relationship between them? Does it indicate some kind of common cause? And, if so, what does that mean for possible preventative measures – even cures?

We'll look at that in Chapter 12.

⊰9⊱

Your Family Tree: A New Ally Against Heart Attacks and Strokes

Meanwhile, let's move on to another group of illnesses that scare the wits out of lots of people – and with good reason, as they are, in fact, the number one causes of death.

These are the thromboses and hypertension (high blood pressure): the silent, invisible killers that abruptly manifest themselves as heart attacks, strokes, cerebral hemorrhages and other cardiovascular catastrophes.

The fit young athlete who drops dead in his thirties with a heart attack . . . the vigorous businessman instantly reduced to a vegetable by a stroke – the sudden, devastating effects of thromboses and hypertension are terrifying enough, but their apparent unpredictability is, perhaps, even worse.

Now, however, that *unpredictability* can be unmasked as the myth that it is, because few other things show up so plainly in a family tree as an above-average risk for thromboses and hypertension. Better still, few other things lend themselves so readily to preventative and corrective action – once you're aware of the risk.

While thromboses and hypertension produce similar results, they differ in origin. So it's best to consider each condition separately.

THROMBOSES: ARE YOU AT RISK?

We'll start with thromboses. What are the things in your family tree that sound a warning of them? The visible effects of previous thromboses, to start with: heart attacks (coronary thromboses and myocardial infarcts), strokes, cerebral hemorrhages, pulmonary thromboses (blood clots in the lungs), deep venous thromboses (such as blood clots in the legs), and so on. Just as a family history of cancer warns of more cancers to come, so a family history of thromboses is the first pointer to more thromboses in the years ahead.

But it's by no means the only one.

There's a whole cluster of illnesses and conditions that, time and again, accompany thromboses through a family tree. No one is quite sure why (although I have some pretty firm ideas), but there's no doubt about the fact itself.

These accomplices of thromboses including diabetes, thyroid disorders and some cancers, particularly gastric cancer and multiple myeloma (cancer of the bones). On the list, too, are multiple sclerosis, our old foes SLE and celiac disease, premature graying, homocystinuria (which we met in Chapter 6), and the dysproteinemias (conditions characterized by raised gamma globulin). And, of course, we mustn't forget our other Chapter 6 acquaintance, hereditary hypercholesterolemia – although its tendency to cause raised cholesterol makes its link with thromboses rather more obvious.

Apart from it and, possibly, homocystinuria, the presence of just one or two of those things in your family tree probably doesn't mean much. But, if several are there – particularly if cases of thromboses have occurred too – the higher-than-average thrombosis risk is certainly present in your family. The risk is even higher for women on the contraceptive pill, and people who have one or more of the *accomplice* conditions themselves.

But what possible link can there be between conditions like those and thromboses? As I said, I have some pretty firm ideas on that – ideas that, once again, flow logically from the hard evidence in a steadily growing number of family trees.

Take another look at the above list of conditions; note particularly that it includes SLE, celiac disease, premature graying and some cancers. We've discussed all of those a number of times before.

And we've seen that a common thread runs through them all – food allergies, especially to milk and grains.

These allergies, you'll remember, impair one's ability to absorb vitamins and minerals from food, leading to serious vitamin-mineral deficiencies. Among the deficiencies so created are those in Vitamins B_6, E, B_3 and C. Each of these, especially the first two, is known to give protection against the risk of abnormal blood clotting. So lower their level in the body and you automatically increase the risk of thromboses.

That, in my view, is the link between thromboses and the conditions listed above. I believe they are all manifestations of the same underlying food allergies and consequent vitamin-mineral deficiencies.

At this point, a very good question may well have entered your mind.

Previously, I've said that such allergies and vitamin-mineral deficiencies can lead to psychiatric symptoms, dementias and cancer. Now I'm saying that, in some families, they can also lead to thromboses. But why? Why don't they produce the same effects in all the families where they occur? The answer is simply this: Each family is different. Different in its diet and lifestyle and particularly in its genetic makeup. Consequently, undetected allergies that produce a certain effect in one family may produce something quite different in another. And in some families, the genetics, diet and lifestyle are such that the blood-clotting mechanisms are one of the first things affected by allergies and vitamin deficiencies.

Other manifestations, as we've seen, usually occur as well: but in those particular families, susceptible people tend to die of heart attacks or strokes before they develop psychiatric symptoms, dementias or cancer.

REDUCING YOUR RISK FOR THROMBOSES

If yours is one of those thrombosis-prone families, what can you do about it?

Fortunately, a great deal.

The first step, of course, is to note exactly what conditions are running in your family. If they were things associated with raised cholesterol and triglycerides, such as thyroid disorders, diabetes, hereditary hypercholesterolemia and the familial hyperlipidemias, you would have your cholesterol and triglyceride levels measured and modify your diet if the levels were up.

Less fatty foods, milk, butter, cheese, eggs, red meat, alcohol and so on – and certainly no cigarettes, especially if your family history includes diabetes or arteriosclerosis (hardening of the arteries). To those "no-nos" add plenty of sensible exercise, plus cholesterol-lowering vitamins such as B_3 and C, and you have the thrombosis-beating prescription for you and your family.

If, on the other hand, your family tree abounded in conditions associated with food allergies and vitamin-mineral deficiencies – particularly SLE, celiac disease, premature graying and gastric cancer – then you would do two things right away.

You would have immediate food allergy tests, especially for grains, eggs, milk and yeast. And you would have your vitamin and mineral levels measured to see if you were low in Vitamins B_6, E, B_3 and C, or the minerals that help those vitamins work more effectively – magnesium, zinc, manganese and selenium.

The chances would be quite high that you or other family members would indeed be allergic to grains, eggs, milk or yeast (or all four), and deficient in those protective vitamins and minerals.

That result would demand a diet totally free of grains, eggs, milk or yeast, and heavy doses of supplementary vitamins and minerals – at least until your body could again absorb them normally from your food. In a fairly short space of time, this should cut your thrombosis risk right down to normal levels.

What if your family tree just showed a history of thromboses, with no accomplice-type disorders? There would still be things you should do. Having tests to determine your levels of cholesterol and triglycerides (types of fat in the blood) would certainly be a worthwhile precaution. And I would definitely recommend that the levels of Vitamins B_6, E, B_3 and C, and their supporting minerals, be checked in yourself and your close relatives.

Please do that even if no other conditions associated with food allergies and consequent vitamin-mineral deficiencies have appeared in your family. They usually do, but not always. In some cases, the food-allergy/vitamin-mineral-deficiency syndrome shows up as thromboses and nothing else.

So, never simply sit back and say, "Oh well, heart attacks and strokes just run in our family." They may indeed seem to do so, but *why* are they running in your family? That's the all-important question doctors so rarely ask – and in your case, unsuspected food allergies and vitamin-mineral deficiencies could well be the answer. If they are, your family's sequence of recurring thromboses can quite easily be brought to an immediate halt.

I firmly believe that not nearly enough attention has been paid to the role of these protective vitamins and minerals in thromboses cases. In fact, I am convinced that all heart-attack victims should have their levels of Vitamins B_6, E, B_3 and C, and important minerals like magnesium, zinc, manganese, calcium and others, tested as a matter of routine. In a high percentage of cases, that would certainly be the key to avoiding further attacks – and the means of preventing them completely in other family members.

And please don't be scared off vitamin- and mineral-level tests by the all-too-frequent medical chorus of "there's no need for them in Western countries; our diets contain plenty of the right vitamins and minerals." It hardly needs pointing out that it doesn't matter how many vitamins and minerals your diet contains if food allergies prevent your body from absorbing them.

It is not what we eat that counts; it is what we absorb.

Indeed, it's very common for people who not only eat good food in abundance, but who take vitamin-mineral supplements as well, to have extremely low vitamin-mineral levels, and all the health problems that flow from them.

Why? Because of their food allergies – most of which have been trumpeting their existence in the family tree for generations.

That's an important point, and worth repeating. If thromboses are running in your family, have your vitamin-mineral levels checked even if no other telltale conditions are present. If that does prove to be your problem – and the chances are high that it will – it's so easy to correct.

You just have your food allergies identified, avoid those foods, take big doses of the relevant vitamins and minerals, get plenty of exercise – and build a new and healthier future for you and your family. Occasionally, however, you do find a family prone to heart attacks and strokes, with no other associated ailments to speak of – and whose members, when tested, show no sign of food allergies or vitamin-mineral deficiencies.

What's likely to be causing the problems in that situation?

If the family really has a *pattern* of heart attacks, strokes and so on, not just a few random (and almost certainly unconnected) cases, there are two likely answers: essential hypertension (high blood pressure without an obvious cause) or some form of hereditary vascular or thrombotic disorder.

HYPERTENSION: HOW TO LESSEN ITS EFFECTS

Let's think for a moment about both candidates, beginning with hypertension – which, as we noted at the start of the chapter, is a major cause of heart attacks, strokes and cerebral hemorrhages.

Sometimes hypertension is the result of other illnesses. Abnormalities of various glands, especially the adrenal and thyroid, can cause it, as can kidney abnormalities, contraceptive pills and a condition called polycythaemia (the opposite of anemia). It can even stem from cardiovascular problems, such as a narrowing of major arteries or blood vessels – a situation that becomes a vicious circle, as the hypertension then worsens the cardiovascular problem, which worsens the hypertension, which. . . .

In such cases, genetic factors usually aren't at work. There's no mystery about the hypertension, and you treat it not only with antihypertensive drugs but also by fixing, wherever possible, the condition that's causing it.

It's quite different with the other kind of hypertension: the one that happens all by itself, with no other condition triggering it off.

This *essential* hypertension occurs in a so-called *benign* form, which can go on for years without doing much damage. However, about 5 percent of cases continue to worsen and eventually enter a *malignant* phase.

When it reaches that point, the condition is a killer.

There are two schools of thought on essential hypertension's origin. The general opinion is that, like height and intelligence, it comes form a combination of several genes and environmental factors. On the other hand, some experts think it's a straightforward autosomal dominant condition, stemming from one rogue gene.

Both schools agree on this: the condition definitely has a genetic element. And it's the first thing you think of when a family contains several unexplained heart attacks, strokes, and other such incidents, with no associated ailments and no evidence of food allergies.

If that sounds like your family, have everybody's blood pressure checked right away. It's among the easiest of medical tests, and in your family's case, it could lead to significant benefits – such as saving lives – in this generation and those to come.

If essential hypertension has been diagnosed in your family, whether recently or in the past, the point to remember is this. The condition has a genetic basis, even if its exact mode of transmission is unclear.

So once you know it's in your family, assume that it's there for the foreseeable future, and from now on, have everyone's blood pressure checked early and regularly.

Anyone with an elevated reading must consider anti-hypertensive drugs, keep their weight down, exercise regularly, give up smoking (which everybody should do anyway), cut back on salt and eat less spices and condiments.

Do those things, and your family tree's warning will almost certainly save you and your family from hyper-tension's effects.

OTHER HEREDITARY CARDIOVASCULAR DISORDERS

Of course, food allergies and hypertension could both get the "not-guilty" verdict in your family. In that case, switch your suspicions immediately to the other heart-attack/stroke promoters – the hereditary vascular or thrombotic disorders.

There are several potential culprits in that category.

It could be hereditary homocystinuria that has never been diagnosed; or hereditary hypercholesterolemia that has similarly escaped identification. It could be one of several hereditary platelet diseases. If the recurring symptom is venous thromboses in the legs, it could be a genetic weakness in the structure of those particular veins.

It could also be polycythaemia, which we met briefly while looking at hypertension. Because this condition makes the blood up to eight times as viscous as normal, it makes people highly at risk for thromboses, too.

Perhaps the family pattern has been one of deaths or disabilities, sometimes occurring in childhood, from strokes or cerebral hemorrhages. In that case, the cause could be berry aneurysms – little balloonlike swellings in blood vessels in the brain that sometimes burst.

Berry aneurysms are hereditary in an autosomal dominant way. However, the mode of transmission of the other conditions is not usually clear.

This latter fact injects a note of difficulty into the investigation. It means that, like hypertension, hereditary vascular and thrombotic disorders rarely form the sort of neat family tree pattern that pinpoints the next person at risk. Their appearance is usually more haphazard, and the risks more widely spread.

Protective measures

If you have reason to suspect that one of the vascular or thrombotic disorders might be running through your family, it's very worthwhile to discuss it with your doctor. Identification is possible and, with most of the disorders, positive protective measures can be undertaken.

Homocystinuria, for example, as you'll remember, frequently responds well to treatment with Vitamin B$_6$. The risks associated with hereditary hypercholesterolemia can be markedly reduced by a fat-free diet. Hereditary platelet diseases, when identified, can be nipped in the bud with anticoagulants. It's not quite as easy, admittedly, with the hereditary structural disorders like berry aneurysms. The best you can say about them is that there are advantages in knowing what you're up against.

If, for example, you have a family history of berry aneurysms, and someone in your family collapses unconscious or suffers a sudden severe headache, you immediately have a very good idea of what's happening. Time won't be wasted on hunting for a diagnosis, and potentially life-saving surgery can be started with minimum delay.

Fortunately, the hereditary structural things are the least common causes of heart attacks, strokes and so on. Most of these killers stem from conditions that can be corrected – and that almost always show up plainly in your family tree.

In fact, the more family trees I see, the more I'm convinced that yours is the best line of defense against thromboses and hypertension. In most cases, it will show you at a glance whether you're an above-average risk. Then it will help you to discover the exact nature of that risk, in plenty of time to eliminate it.

Before it eliminates you.

❧10❧

Compile Your Family Tree and Stay Sane

In a previous Chapter I suggested that cancer is possibly the most feared illness of all. That may be so; but, if it has a rival for that unenviable position, psychosis or mental illness must surely be it. Probably that's because of the age-old stigma that clings to mental illness . . . the feeling that it is somehow *different* from all other disorders . . . the impression it gives of stripping away one's humanity, and of having no observable or recognizable cause.

Even today, there's a widespread belief that if people become mentally ill, they must have been "funny" or "strange" all along. And if they recover, many will still look at them with suspicion, and regard them as unreliable for the rest of their lives.

Popular phrases continue to reflect this attitude, and to reinforce it in people's minds. Calling a psychiatric hospital a "funny farm" is a prime example. So is saying that someone has "gone round the bend," with its suggestion that he or she has passed out of the normal human scene into some new and alien landscape.

But uninformed lay people are not the only ones, I believe, who perpetuate the fear and misunderstanding that hang like a mist around mental illness. I believe much orthodox psychiatry adds to it – by insisting that mental illness is always the result of strains, stresses and conflicts in one's environment or upbringing.

None of us had a perfect upbringing. And we've all experienced strains, stresses and conflicts. So, if some of us crack up under such influences, while most people survive them, the clear implication is that we are somehow *weaker* than the hardier folk around us.

Spoken or unspoken, that's a very common attitude in our society. It flows quite logically from the generally accepted view of the causes of mental illness. And by taking a further swipe at their already battered self-esteem, it is enormously destructive to people who are mentally ill.

It is also totally untrue.

THE PHYSICAL BASIS OF MENTAL ILLNESS

I don't accept for a moment that the main cause of mental illness is unresolved strains, stresses and conflicts. I believe that mental illness almost always has a physical basis – and that, in the great majority of cases, the physical basis stands out like a beacon in the family tree.

That's not to say that strains, stresses and conflicts play no part in mental illness. They do, of course; but the real question is: Why do only some of the people who experience them become mentally ill? The answer, I believe, is that those people have an underlying physical condition that makes them much more susceptible to unresolved stress. As I indicated a moment ago, that condition is almost always a hereditary one, or the result of hereditary factors.

So, if you're worried about mental illness striking you or your loved ones, get cracking now on your family tree.

The value of doing so has been underlined many times in our earlier chapters. Remember Jack? First, they thought he had a brain tumor. Then a nervous breakdown. Then schizophrenia. Until his family tree unmasked the wheat allergy that was really causing his baffling symptoms.

Remember Ellen? Diagnosed as schizophrenic. Given shock treatment without results. Fruitlessly dosed to the eyeballs with tranquilizers and antidepressants. Then set free when her family tree pointed to her autoimmune disease.

Remember Pat? Averaging nine months a year in psychiatric hospitals. Getting every treatment modern psychiatry could offer, from drugs to shock treatment to sleep therapy. Finding relief only when her food allergies were uncovered by her family tree.

Remember Coralie? Facing psychosurgery as the "only hope" (so she was told) of relieving her profound depression. However, it melted away quite obediently once her family tree alerted us to her SLE.

Glance back, too, at those earlier chapters and recall the Woodbridge and Ransome families, Valerie, and Susan and Nancy. They all had profound psychiatric symptoms that had resisted traditional treatment. Yet they all improved tremendously when we followed the lead given by their family trees – in every instance they were loaded with conditions like bowel cancer, arthritis, pernicious anemia, vitamin deficiencies and SLE.

Now, it's time to test your memory. A growing body of evidence suggests strongly that all those conditions frequently have a common cause. What is it?

Did you say grain allergies? Go to the top of the class, and give yourself a bonus mark if you can anticipate the conclusion I'm about to draw.

It's not a conclusion that will have orthodox psychiatrists bounding to their feet with wild applause and cheers. Nevertheless, here it is.

In the light of the cases we've just reviewed, and perhaps 1500 others like them that I've treated, I'm convinced that psychiatric symptoms almost always have physical causes. The most common of these is gluten sensitivity, or in plain words, grain allergies.

As I said, orthodox psychiatrists will be somewhat less than happy with that conclusion. Traditionally, they divided psychoses into two groups: *organic* and *affective*.

Organic psychoses, as the name implies, are those that stem from an organic or physical cause. *Affective psychoses*, on the other hand, are those that spring entirely from stress factors in the patient's environment or upbringing.

Or so the theory runs. What I'm saying is that *affective* psychoses, for all intents and purposes, don't exist. I believe that *organic* psychoses are the only kind there are – and grain allergies are their most common cause.

If I'm right, two implications immediately follow.

First, psychosis victims are no more to blame for their condition than are flu victims. So any basis for attaching a stigma to mental illness is instantly and permanently destroyed

Second, the vast majority of psychoses can be predicted and prevented – or treated, if they've already occurred – by means of the family tree.

Which, believe me, is a much more humane and pleasant approach than battering people with shock treatment, psychosurgery and massive doses of antidepressants. It's also a lot more effective.

FIGHTING PSYCHOSES WITH YOUR FAMILY TREE

So, let's suppose that you do have a psychotic relative or two, and you're concerned about your chance of going the same way. How can you use your family tree to make sure you don't?

Well, if grain allergies are, as I believe, the most common cause of psychoses, you obviously start by looking for their footprints in your family tree. And after the last three chapters, you shouldn't have much trouble in spotting them.

Remember?

Gastric cancer, frequent viral infections, hyperactivity in children, diabetes, pellagra. Plus that grain-allergy-linked cluster of autoimmune diseases – disorders of the thyroid, adrenal, parathyroid and pituitary glands. And, perhaps most important of all, SLE and other connective tissue disorders, celiac disease and pernicious anemia – or, if those three have never been diagnosed, their symptoms and signs: vague aches and pains, arthritis, butterfly rash on the face, burning easily in the sun, prematurely gray hair, early baldness, chronic indigestion and frequent diarrhea.

If you have some of those things in your family tree, as well as psychoses, the chances are very high that the psychoses are the result of grain allergies, and the malabsorption of essential vitamins and minerals that the grain allergies cause.

In that case, you can start celebrating. Your mentally ill relatives can almost certainly be cured swiftly and easily on a strict grain-free diet and hefty doses of relevant vitamins and minerals. So don't waste a day. Have them tested for grain allergies and vitamin-mineral deficiencies just as soon as you can. And then go a step further, and have the same tests done on every other family member in the firing line.

Who are they? First, those who have any of the diseases I have just mentioned. Second, those who don't, but are in an X-linked relationship with those who do – that is, symptom-free girls with an affected mother, father, maternal grandparent or paternal grandmother, and symptom-free males with an affected mother or maternal grandparent.

The second category is important, because there's growing evidence that the genetic predisposition for nearly all these grain-allergy-based conditions could be X-linked. So, for symptom-free people with an X-linkage to someone with symptoms, grain-allergy tests are a very wise precaution.

While it might be easy to cure grain-allergy psychoses, it's much better not to get them at all.

OTHER ALLERGIES AND PSYCHOSES

Extremely important though they are, grains are by no means the only allergies to cause psychiatric symptoms. Milk, for instance, is right in there behind them. Almost as common, too, are legume allergies – their devastating role in causing psychoses is only just becoming recognized.

Fortunately, when allergists test you for grain allergies, they normally run tests for many other food allergies at the same time. So, if milk or legume allergies rather than grain allergies are behind your problems, the tests will still pick them up – and start you on the road to prediction, prevention and cure. Legume allergies, incidentally, are the reason why every psychosis-plagued family should have food-allergy tests, even if no grain-allergy signs are appearing in their members. Legume allergies frequently leave little or no trace of their presence in the family tree – apart from recurring psychoses. Food-allergy tests are often the only way to pick them up.

But what exactly are *legumes*, you ask? Technically, they're any sort of plant that fixes nitrogen in a nodule under the soil. Those that we eat include soybeans, peanuts, beans, lentils and peas. And if you're sufficiently allergic to them, especially the first two, they'll not only cause psychiatric symptoms themselves but will cut your vitamin-mineral absorption to a very low level indeed. One quite low enough to cause all the classic symptoms of schizophrenia – inappropriate moods, disordered thinking, delusions, paranoia (feelings of persecution) and hallucinations.

Hereditary food allergies, then, come immediately to mind whenever you see a pattern of psychosis running through a family. But such a pattern can also occur without any allergies at all. In such cases, other hereditary factors are usually the culprits; and with a bit of sharp-eyed sleuthing, they too can be seen at work in the family tree.

These factors fall under the general heading of hereditary inborn errors of metabolism. The fact that they cause psychiatric disorders has been recognized only in fairly recent years. The main types of psychoses they produce have been called pyroluria and porphyria. While these conditions have been identified only recently, it seems that several historically prominent people may well have suffered from them.

PYROLURIA: TWO FAMOUS SUFFERERS

The evidence suggests, for instance, that both Charles Darwin and Emily Dickinson, the poet, had pyroluria.

Despite their brilliant achievements, each of these outstanding people had episodes of deep depression, mood swings, inner tension, rapid pulse, severe headaches and nervous exhaustion. As their lives went on, both changed from sociable folk into semi-recluses, with a growing fear of getting involved with anyone outside their family circles. And as this change progressed, their handwriting altered and became harder to read.

All those things are typical symptoms of pyroluria. Darwin had several others, including abdominal pain, nausea and insomnia, plus a feature very often found in pyrolurics – coarse eyebrows. It is not known whether Emily had those particular pointers to the disease, but she did have another one – a pale, lustrous, china-doll complexion.

Pyroluria is surprisingly common. One study estimates that 10 percent of the total population suffers from it, while 30 percent of people hospitalized for schizophrenia actually have pyroluria. It's certainly a hereditary complaint, but the manner of its transmission is not yet clear. Sometimes it seems to be autosomal dominant, sometimes autosomal recessive and sometimes X-linked.

This uncertainty makes it harder to tell which people within a family are at risk, and many more family trees are needed before the question can be resolved. So, if your family tree happens to contain pyroluria, it could ultimately benefit many families besides your own.

How can you tell if it does contain pyroluria?

You look for an interesting combination of symptoms and signs – some of which we have already seen occurring in Charles and Emily. Then you look for people with *schizoaffective* disorders. Their schizophrenic symptoms are accompanied by a deep and profound depression, or by mood swings that lift them out of the blues into an exaggerated elation, only to plunge them back again.

You also look for people who suffer from feelings of tension: the constant tiredness of nervous exhaustion, rapid pulse, severe headaches or pains in the lower left abdomen, creaking joints while still teenagers.

Then you scan your ranks for people with coarse eyebrows or white dots in the fingernails. People who can't recall their dreams or claim they never dream (sounds strange, but, as we'll see soon, an important clue). And people with cancer – the combination of cancer and schizoaffective disorders in a family is a strong pointer to pyroluria.

Another characteristic of pyroluric families is a high incidence of boy babies being miscarried or stillborn, or born with severe or fatal birth defects. So a strong indication of pyroluria is all-girl families, with one or more of the girls developing psychiatric symptoms in her late teens.

As we've seen before, the symptoms listed above don't all have to occur in the one person. A typical pyroluric family tree might have some people with schizoaffective disorders, others with cancer and others with (say) depression and headaches. Or there could be schizoaffective disorders in some folk, while others have creaking joints and abdominal pains or rapid pulse and nervous exhaustion. There could be a couple of all-girl families with teenage psychiatric sufferers and a sprinkling of the other symptoms in grandparents, parents, uncles, aunts and cousins.

If your family tree looks like any of those, pyroluria is probably not only the common link between all your problems, but the direct cause of the psychiatric symptoms.

And once you suspect that, you can cut through the time-wasting, fruitless procedure that happens all too often – trying to treat the psychiatric symptoms while ignoring their cause. You can get right to the cause itself and treat it: Pyroluria, fortunately, is easy to establish, easy to treat and easy to cure.

The test for pyroluria is to see whether the urine contains chemical substances known as kryptopyrroles. If it does, the diagnosis is positive. It's as simple as that – and the treatment is equally simple.

The excretion of kryptopyrroles drains the body of Vitamin B_6 and zinc. It's the loss of these vital substances that causes the psychiatric symptoms – and that strange feature of not being able to recall dreams or not dreaming at all. The treatment is appropriate doses of Vitamin B_6 and zinc. And the response is usually quite spectacular. Most patients make a swift and complete recovery, as long as the Vitamin B_6 and zinc are maintained and increased in times of extra stress.

The next step, of course, is prediction and prevention. Because of the uncertainty of pyroluria's mode of transmission, all near relatives of affected people should be considered at risk – especially those who have any of pyroluria's accompanying telltale symptoms. Urine tests will then quickly establish whether the risk is becoming a reality.

If it is, regular doses of Vitamin B_6 and zinc will, in most cases, permanently prevent the psychiatric symptoms from appearing; and, if any of the other symptoms are present, lead to a very considerable improvement in them as well.

Of course, before those gratifying cures and preventions can occur, the pyroluria has to be identified. If your doctor thinks he's dealing with just another schizophrenia, no progress will be made. Here's where your family tree is vital – to point straight to the real culprit and prevent a frustrating welter of wild goose chasing.

PORPHYRIA: THE ROYAL PSYCHOSIS

Pyroluria, you'll recall, may have affected Charles Darwin and Emily Dickinson. Porphyria, its near but much rarer relative, may be nearly as notable a psychosis in that royalty has probably been among its victims.

King George III, for instance, is now believed to have been one of them. You'll recall from your history lessons that he ruled England from 1760 to 1820, and that from about 1811 he was trapped in a hopeless haze of madness. The record of his symptoms has convinced some researchers that porphyria was his problem.

Porphyria is an autosomal dominant complaint, but fortunately for the British royal family, George III's son, the Duke of Kent, didn't get it, despite his 50 percent chance of doing so. Because he escaped the faulty gene himself, he couldn't pass it on to his daughter, Queen Victoria. Porphyria was consequently bred out of the current British royal line – although Queen Victoria did cause a bit of strife by bequeathing hemophilia to some of her male descendants.

That, however, is another story.

Porphyria shows up in the family tree in a number of subtle, yet definite, ways. To start with, sufferers are linked together in an autosomal dominant pattern. Their psychiatric symptoms often follow the taking of certain drugs – especially barbiturates, penicillin, sulfa drugs, the contraceptive pill (because of its estrogen) and chloroquin (the antimalarial drug), or appear after the patient has been on a high protein, low carbohydrate diet.

Another distinctive sign is that the psychosis usually shows up fairly early in life, typically before the age of thirty. It's frequently accompanied by neurological symptoms such as foot drop – which, as the name implies, means you have trouble lifting your feet and tend to drag them as you walk. Epilepsy often goes along with porphyria, as do abdominal pains, nausea, vomiting and constipation.

The abdominal pains, in fact, can be so severe that many porphyrics are subjected to exploratory abdominal operations, and sometimes more than one. These operations, of course, reveal nothing. All too often, the patients are then scornfully called "neurotics" or "malingerers," with the implication that they are imagining or even faking the pain.

Eventually, if they're lucky, the correct diagnosis is made.

So, if mental illness has been recurring in your family, and your family tree doesn't seem to point to allergies or pyroluria, take another look at it. Are the sufferers linked together in an autosomal dominant pattern? Did some of them develop psychiatric symptoms when they were dieting – or after taking the contraceptive pill or one of the other drugs listed above? Did their psychoses appear in their teens or twenties? Were the women psychotic once a month, before their periods? And did any of them also have a dragging or shuffling gait, epilepsy, abdominal problems and/or abdominal operations?

If so, porphyria is your number one suspect.

Once you've arrived at that conclusion, you can make swift progress. The first step is arranging tests to confirm the family tree's diagnosis. After that, treatment and prevention can begin.

Porphyria is, as I said before, a hereditary metabolic disorder that results in increased porphyrins (a type of chemical) in the urine. The basic treatment is a diet high in carbohydrates and low in fat and proteins. This diet, the opposite of many popular slimming regimes, counteracts the metabolic malfunctions and gets the body chemistry working more normally.

As a result, most people with porphyria can look forward to living a normal or near normal life – as long as they avoid the drugs mentioned above and don't embark on a high protein, low carbohydrate, slimming diet.

Thanks to the family tree, moreover, those in line for porphyria can look forward to not developing it at all. We've already seen that porphyria is an autosomal dominant complaint. That makes it pretty easy to predict who in the family is at risk. The next step is fairly obvious: a high carbohydrate, low fat and low protein diet for all of them.

If that diet is continued on a regular basis and the harmful drugs are avoided, the potential porphyria, in most cases, simply won't develop.

Schizophrenia: why it may have a genetic base

So far, we've talked about psychiatric conditions that produce schizophrenialike symptoms, but aren't really what doctors understand by the term *schizophrenia*. They are very often mistaken for it; but they aren't, in terms of current medical terminology, schizophrenia in the true sense.

Consequently, while many, or even most, cases of so-called schizophrenia are really allergic conditions or hereditary metabolic disorders, a significant minority remains that doesn't appear to fit into either category. These can be called the true schizophrenias. Is your family tree of any value in such cases? It certainly is – it could help to unravel the mystery of these schizophrenias, establish their cause and lead to a cure.

For decades, the cause of schizophrenia has been the elusive target of dozens of researchers. They have wandered down all sorts of hypothetical pathways, flirted with viruses, pondered long over environmental possibilities – and switched at last to what I'm sure is the right track.

The genetic one.

Right now, in fact, the search for a genetic basis to schizophrenia is being hotly pursued. What touched it off was a fascinating series of studies that seem to have dealt the environmental theory a final and fatal blow.

It became obvious some time ago that schizophrenia tends to cluster in families. "There you are," said the environmentalists. "Obviously, the influence of a schizophrenic parent or sibling makes others go the same way." That sounded logical, but some researchers weren't convinced. They embarked on long-term studies of what happens when the children of schizophrenics are brought up elsewhere, while others stay at home.

Several such studies have now been conducted, and the results are quite conclusive. You're much more likely to get schizophrenia if you're directly related to someone who already has it. The children who are adopted at birth and brought up away from their parents still show a high incidence of the disease. Conversely, those brought up in a family with schizophrenics, but who aren't related to them, rarely become schizophrenic themselves. Their risk is no higher than that of the community at large.

In a 1982 comment on these studies, the *British Journal of Psychiatry* said that the genetic theory for the cause of schizophrenia now "rests on more secure grounds" than any other. What is not yet known, however, is the mode of transmission, and precisely what it is that is inherited and causes the psychosis. That's why your family tree could be so important. The only way of determining those two points is to get more and more family trees – and yours could be just the one to provide a vital clue.

Additional evidence for schizophrenia's genetic basis has already come from a number of studies of family trees. Some of these have shown definite genetic markers accompanying schizophrenia through a family. This means that whatever was causing the schizophrenia was almost certainly being carried on the same gene as the markers themselves. Hairy fingers, hair coloring and type, ear shape, earlobe form, eye coloring, length of fingers, being left- or right-handed and the way the tongue curled were some of the markers identified.

Another study showed five albino people in one family, all suffering from a form of schizophrenia. The probability of a genetic linkage in this case was felt to be very strong. Other studies have produced rather more esoteric markers, such as blood groups, sensitivity to particular pathology tests and the presence of group-specific antigens.

So, in this sense, schizophrenia is rather like cancer. It's an area where ordinary people could provide the all-important research breakthrough – simply by compiling their family trees.

MANIC-DEPRESSIVE PSYCHOSES

Moving away from the schizophrenic group of illnesses, we come to the next common mental disorders – the manic-depressive psychoses. It was one of these, you'll remember, that the Woodbridge family had. And from them we learned two very important things. Manic-depressive psychosis is X-linked in many families and, if yours is one, your family tree is your surest path to prediction, prevention and cure.

When you've compiled your family tree, it's fairly easy to tell whether any manic-depressive illness in your family is X-linked. If the sufferers are joined in an X-linked relationship, that's very significant. And, if any of them share the same X-linked genetic markers, the case is doubly strong.

Such markers include red-green color blindness, Xg negative blood group, and (while they're not strictly X-linked) such physical characteristics as hair, eye and complexion color. They can also include hereditary metabolic disorders and the whole range of familial autoimmune endocrine diseases, the predisposition for which appears to be X-linked in many cases.

While all those markers are important for establishing X-linkage – which in turn establishes who in the family is at risk – it's the last two groups that are important for treatment and prevention.

All of them are treatable conditions. And you'll recall the principle we established in Chapter 4. Look for treatable X-linked conditions that are running along with the manic-depressive illness – or with any other serious illness, for that matter. Treat them, and you'll treat the major problem, because both are manifestations of the same underlying genetic disorder.

What's more, you rarely find an X-linked manic-depressive psychosis that isn't accompanied by a treatable X-linked condition. That's been my experience, anyway; and it means that the family tree has provided the healing clue in nearly every X-linked manic-depressive psychosis I've ever seen.

Are there people with manic-depressive psychosis in your family? Then get started right away on your family tree. And take another look at the Woodbridge case history in Chapter 4.

What the family tree did for them (and at least 200 other manic-depressive sufferers I've seen), it can do for you.

MISCELLANEOUS MENTAL DISORDERS

The various forms of schizophrenia-type illnesses, porphyria, pyroluria, and the manic-depressive psychoses account for the great bulk of mental disorders. There are others, of course, but they're fairly rare – in some of those, too, the family tree is of real value.

Huntington's chorea, which we examined in the last chapter, is frequently mistaken at first for a psychosis. However, a glance at the family tree dispels that idea and tells you the unpleasant truth. It can't suggest a cure, unfortunately, because at the moment there isn't one; but at least it shows you what you're up against and how to get it out of the family . . . by indicating who's at risk and who shouldn't have children.

Sometimes, young people (ages from 10 to 25) arrive on the psychiatrist's doorstep with an apparent psychosis or dementia, plus a slight tremor. That could suggest all sorts of things, until the family tree indicates that it's happened before in the patient's family, and in an autosomal recessive pattern.

You then think of Wilson's disease, a condition caused by deposits of copper in the liver and brain, resulting in cirrhosis of both organs. To treat it, you give the patient what are called *chelating* agents, to get rid of the copper, and add heavy doses of Vitamin C and zinc. The condition can be treated if caught early enough – where the family tree helps, by pointing in the right direction and saving a lot of time hunting around for a diagnosis.

Despite all I've said in this chapter, I'm not suggesting that every single psychosis has a genetic base. There are quite a number of psychotic conditions that appear, on the surface anyway, to be totally unrelated to hereditary factors. These include psychoses caused by drugs such as LSD, by unusual reactions to therapeutic drugs, and by diseases such as epilepsy, brain tumors and infections such as syphilis.

Sleep deprivation can bring on paranoid symptoms. And it's quite common for a severe reactive depression to follow bereavement, job loss or other personal trauma. All these seem to be nonhereditary and likely to happen to anyone, given the circumstances.

It would appear that, in such cases the family tree won't help. And yet . . . I wonder.

The question still arises – why do some people become psychotic in those circumstances, while others don't? What makes some people more susceptible? Is it something in their genetic makeup – or some hereditary allergy, vitamin deficiency or metabolic defect?

If it were the latter, the family tree would usually reveal it. And knowing about it would greatly increase the chances of a cure. That's why I think a family tree should always be drawn up in psychiatric cases, even if the condition seems to be a nonhereditary one.

And in the major mental illnesses – the schizophrenic group, pyroluria, porphyria and manic-depression – the value of the family tree is beyond doubt: that is, if you want to discover and treat the causes of the psychosis. Not just its symptoms.

❊11❊

How to Present Your Family Tree to Your Doctor

By now, hopefully, you're convinced that your family tree can be one of the greatest medical assets you can possess. But there's another key person in your healing process that may not, at first, totally share your convictions. And that's your doctor.

Not all doctors, I hasten to add, are "Doubting Thomases" about family trees. Indeed, a majority will see their significance at a glance. But just in case yours is one of the minority, let's consider how to present your family tree to him or her: to ensure you get maximum benefit from it, and to make him or her a wholehearted convert to the family tree cause.

Fortunately, in my experience, once doctors really take a look at a well-presented family tree, their conversations tend to follow almost automatically. So the first step to achieving that happy result – which will help both your doctor and you – is to see that your family tree is properly drawn up.

Don't draw it upside down

When I say "properly drawn up," I mean drawn up to the standards we established in Chapter 6. Everyone in his or her right generation. Squares for males, circles for females. Relevant sicknesses and conditions clearly marked and keyed.

A sloppily drawn family tree will only confuse your doctor and kill interest on the spot. Doctors are busy people and don't have time to decode puzzles. I've even seen family trees drawn upside down, with the great-grandparents at the bottom and the proband at the top.

Just as an upside-down book is hard to read, so is an upside-down family tree.

But all these traps are easy to avoid. Simply follow the basic rules in Chapter 6, and you'll have no trouble in drawing up a family tree that's clear, informative and easy to read.

THE NEXT STEP: AROUSING INTEREST

A doctor who is not yet switched on to the family tree approach may blink when you proudly slap your master-piece down on the desk. That's when you have to move quickly, before the blinks turn into a haze of bewilderment and disinterest.

Start by telling him or her just *why* you've brought the family tree. Using the knowledge you've gained from this book, tell your doctor *why* you think the conditions listed in your family tree may be linked with your symptoms.

Emphasize what seem to be the *relevant* things, and why you think they're relevant. Indicate any *categories* of illness that appear to be running in the family – cancers, neurological problems, heart and blood vessel disorders, and so on. (of course, if you've found enough information, you may have each category on a separate family tree).

Point out any *patterns* that there are – clusters of autoimmune diseases, for instance, or the telltale signs of food allergies. And if you can see the *types of transmission* involved – autosomal dominant, X-linked recessive, etc. – and who is at risk for what illness, be sure to emphasize that too.

At this point, any doubtful hazes should be quickly fading from your doctor's eyes. He or she is most likely to be leaning forward and studying your family tree with very real interest indeed.

After all, every conscientious person wants to do a better job, and doctors are no exception. And by this stage, your doctor will be realizing that your family tree can help him or her to do an even better job of caring for you and your family.

PICKING THE SERIOUS **10** PERCENT

To start with, it will help to overcome the busy general practitioner's greatest worry: the ever-present risk of not recognizing a potentially serious illness.

At least 90 percent of a GP's patients have relatively trivial complaints – minor infections, tension headaches, coughs, colds and flu. And when you're seeing those things all day and every day, it's very easy to miss something really serious – especially as it frequently starts off looking just like another case of day-to-day trivia.

For every GP, the trick is to pick the fewer than 10 percent of patients who do have a major problem. Here the family tree is the doctor's more effective ally.

For instance, if you have a bad headache, your doctor is much less likely to dismiss it as meaningless if your family tree contains berry aneurysms (Chapter 9).

If you're depressed and losing weight, he or she will investigate you far more thoroughly if gastric cancer has occurred a few times in your family.

If you complain of painful indigestion, you won't just be given a simple antacid if your family tree is full of heart attacks and associated ailments.

In other words, a family tree can positively shout that, in many people, seemingly minor symptoms may be the start of devastating illness. It immediately alerts the doctor to the possibility. Then it tells him or her the relevant tests to do and, as we've seen before, greatly reduces the chance of a wrong diagnosis being made, or a potentially major problem being overlooked.

Of the 10 percent of GP patients who are seriously ill, the problems of a small proportion are initially unrecognized each year. And the rarer and more dangerous their condition, the more likely it is to be missed.

Your family tree can help to ensure that you and your relatives are not among the missed ones. That is not only great for you, but for your doctor as well – anything that helps to spot a serious illness that might otherwise have slipped through will be welcomed with open arms.

HELP YOUR DOCTOR NOT TO HURT YOU

Another area in which your family tree can be helpful is that dignified by the name of *iatrogenic* illnesses.

These are not, as might be supposed, illnesses caused by exotic bacteria or viruses. The name covers a whole host of disorders caused, or made worse, by the drugs doctors are prescribing to cure other ailments. An extreme sensitivity to penicillin, leading to severe allergic reactions or even death, is a familiar example; but there are lots more, and a great number of them would be revealed to your doctor by a detailed family tree.

Take SLE, for instance. When it's present but unrecognized in a family, it can create all sorts of complications when doctors are trying to treat other illnesses. Let's imagine that you have high blood pressure, arthritis and (without knowing it) SLE. Your doctor's first, and totally correct, move would be to lower the blood pressure with antihypertensive drugs.

Unfortunately, however, the most commonly used antihypertensives are likely to make the SLE worse. So, quite unwittingly, the doctor would be doing the wrong thing for you by applying what would normally be the right line of treatment.

Or, if you, with your unsuspected SLE, had a severe infection, your doctor might attack it with penicillin or sulphonamides. That would be unfortunate, too, because both types of drug, usually so appropriate in that situation, are also likely to aggravate the SLE, and leave you worse off than you were before.

On the other hand, if your doctor had your family tree and saw SLE or its signs there, with you in the firing line for it, he or she would know precisely what to do. You would be investigated and treated for SLE, your real problem, while your blood pressure or infection was brought under control by alternative drugs.

Many more potential iatrogenic problems can be headed off quite easily by a family tree. If mold allergies are revealed there, the doctor would know to be careful in prescribing antibiotics. If your family tree warns of a hereditary sensitivity to certain anesthetics, that information could be life-saving if someone in the family needs to have an operation.

Iatrogenic illness is a growing problem in medicine today. The widespread use of family trees could be a major step toward overcoming it.

SAVE YOUR DOCTOR'S TIME, AND YOU'LL BENEFIT

As well as helping your doctor to be more effective, your family tree can make his or her job easier by saving valuable time. Most doctors would love to obtain a detailed medical history of their patients' families, because they do realize how such information would help them: but with a crowded waiting room of impatient patients out there, they simply haven't the time to do it.

However, when you bring them that vital information, all carefully researched and well laid out, that's a whole new ball game. They don't have to spend time asking you vital questions about your family. They can plunge straight into helping you, with the way ahead clearly signposted for them.

Suddenly, you're not "just another patient," but someone who's gone to considerable trouble to help them to help you, to make their job easier and more rewarding – maybe even to give them some new insights into various illnesses. That will be genuinely appreciated, because doctors are human too. And in return, you'll get more informed (and hence better) treatment, better diagnosis and better follow-up.

Perhaps, most important, you'll sow the seeds of a healthier future. Even if you're quite free from them at the moment, you'll alert your doctor to the illnesses you're most at risk for. And you'll give him or her the chance to guard you against them. Prevention, as we've observed before, is many times better than the most effective cure.

OTHER DOCTORS, OTHER PLACES, OTHER FAMILY MEMBERS

Sometimes, of course, illnesses don't give you time to practice preventative medicine. They strike suddenly out of the blue: often at times and in places where your own doctor is unavailable. Then your life hinges on the skills of a doctor who knows nothing about you or your genetic makeup. These are the times when the margin for error is smallest – and when your family tree can play a crucial role.

Suppose, for example, that you collapse and are rushed to a hospital. It's the weekend, and your family doctor can't be contacted. Any one of a dozen things could be wrong: but if a relative takes your family tree to the hospital with you, it could well give the vital diagnostic clue that could make the difference between life and death.

It may, for instance, point to berry aneurysms in your family, or a high risk for cerebral hemorrhages or strokes, or diabetes, suggesting that you're in a diabetic coma.

Whatever it is, your family tree can give any doctor an immediate and intimate picture of your likely problems. And, of course, warn of any dangers associated with treatment or surgery, such as sensitivity to drugs or anesthetics, or conditions like hemophilia (uncontrollable bleeding).

For these reasons, if there are conditions like diabetes, thromboses, hypertension, berry aneurysms, drug sensitivity, hemophilia, homocystinuria and so on in your family, I think it's a good idea to take your family tree with you if you're going away – especially if you're going overseas. Then, if a crisis does arise, you have something that can say a lot to a doctor when you can't; and cut right across language barriers in the process.

The ability of a family tree to speak on your behalf is, by the way, a good reason for drawing one up as early as possible – before accidents, strokes, dementia, deafness or other handicaps make it difficult or impossible for you to communicate with your doctor.

And, of course, it's not only on your behalf that your family tree can speak, but also on behalf of your relatives. As we've emphasized many times in this book, the benefits of a family tree overflow from you to all the members of your family. And that's especially valuable when they're in the care of a doctor other than your local GP.

If your family doctor does get new light and guidance on your problems from your family tree, and you have relatives with similar problems, then a real breakthrough has been achieved. Maybe those relatives are just living apart from you. Perhaps they're actually in hospitals or institutions. Either way, be sure to tell your doctor about them. Then he or she can share the good news with their doctors – and so the family tree's healing insights will spread.

HOW YOUR FAMILY TREE CAN HELP MANKIND

It might be that your family tree's value will extend far beyond your distant relatives. It could even finish up being of tremendous benefit to all mankind.

The more family trees we get to study, the more we'll learn about the genetic and allergic factors involved in hosts of different illnesses – cancer, schizophrenia, heart disease, dementia, MS and many more. And every advance in our knowledge will hasten the day when all these diseases are finally conquered.

Perhaps your family tree will be the one to provide a vital clue. Perhaps your family doctor will see something in it that you don't, and realize that you've not only helped him or her to help you, but that you've also helped millions of people throughout the world.

In that case, your family tree will be sent to the appropriate research institute. Whether or not that happens, I'd like to see your family tree myself. I want to collect as many as possible, because I believe that, when enough are available for research, the exciting healing possibilities we're seeing in this book will be confirmed as facts. When that happens, freedom will come to millions of folk who are now sentenced to pain, misery, despair and death. Wouldn't it be something if your family tree helped the world to attain that goal?

It certainly would. So please send a copy of your family tree (not the original) to:

Dr. C. M. Reading
P.O. Box 587
DEE WHY. N.S.W. 2099
AUSTRALIA.

PART THREE

The Big Mysteries: New Clues from Family Trees

All advances in medicine – indeed, in science generally – begin when someone formulates a theory, usually on the basis of something he or she has observed.

In the last section, I'm going to formulate a few theories on the real nature of some very nasty illnesses, based on my observations of some startling family trees.

The theories are, admittedly, speculative. However, if they prove to be valid, we'll be able to treat, predict and prevent things like Down's Syndrome, Alzheimer's disease, some forms of cancer, muscular dystrophy, motor neuron disease and multiple sclerosis, much more effectively than is now possible.

No one with a personal or professional interest in any of those illnesses can, I believe, afford to ignore these family trees. Examine them with me now – I think you'll agree.

❖12❖

Down's Syndrome and Other Illnesses: Some Significant Family Trees

All through this book, we've seen how family trees can throw new light on the causes of cancer, psychoses, dementia and many other serious illnesses.

In these last two chapters, I want to look at some especially interesting family trees that underline what we've been saying in earlier pages, and at some others that go even further and open up exciting new areas for research and speculation.

I want to suggest, too, that your family tree could be just as exciting, just as thought-provoking and just as valuable for research as any in this book.

With that in mind, let's start by looking at four extremely serious conditions – Down's Syndrome (mongolism), leukemia, lymphoma (bowel cancer) and Alzheimer's disease (the dementia that we met in Chapter 8).

A SINISTER LINK

It has long been recognized that there's some sort of link between the four. The brothers and sisters and other near relatives of people with Alzheimer's disease have a higher-than-normal incidence of leukemia, lymphoma and Down's Syndrome. Down's Syndrome children themselves face an even greater risk of leukemia – one far above the community average – and of those who dodge it, a large proportion develop Alzheimer's disease in early adult life.

That much is well known and documented. What is missing is an explanation for the link: some identifiable common factor, also present in such families, that could tell us why the four conditions go together, and even hint at a common cause.

On the basis of some of my family trees, and the investigations they led me to make, I think I know what that link, and possible common cause, could be. I'm a long way from offering hard scientific proof, but I'm convinced that the ideas provoked by these family trees should be followed up with urgent and concentrated research.

Some of the family trees are fairly simple. One, on its own probably wouldn't have suggested much to me, but what I find significant is that these, and several others I have, are all saying the same thing.

THE HOPKINS FAMILY: FOUR GENERATIONS OF MISFORTUNE

The first one (*Figure 30*) is that of the Hopkins family. Young Craig Hopkins is a Down's Syndrome child. His mother, Jill, has lymphoma, or bowel cancer. Her father, Jack, now deceased, also had bowel cancer. And Jack's mother, Florence, died of breast cancer.

Not a happy picture, you'll agree. But what could cause such a four-generation pattern of misfortune? Well, if you remember Chapter 7, our cancer chapter, you'll recall that this sort of cancer family picture is almost always accompanied by something else – autoimmune disease – including, and especially, celiac disease and its basis, severe grain allergies.

Was that the problem – and perhaps even the cause of the cancer – in the Hopkins family? It was a bit late to find out with long-dead Jack and Florence, but Jill was still around and, although seriously ill, was putting up a great fight against her bowel cancer. So I had some tests run on her. The results were extremely significant.

Jill was highly allergic to gluten, one of the components of grain; and she was full of autoimmune antibodies. Now, not everyone with marked allergies to grains or

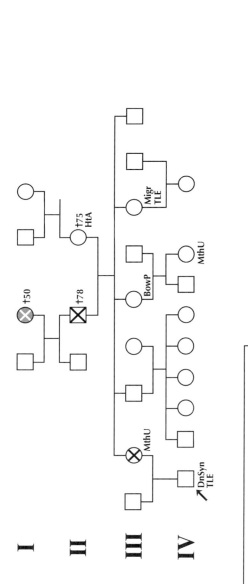

FIGURE 30: the Hopkins family

Three cancers in three generations: Did that point to celiac disease and grain allergies? And if so, what bearing did it have on the Down's Syndrome child's condition?

Bow P = Bowel problems
Dn Syn = Down's syndrome
Ht A   = Heart attack (coronary occlusion)

Migr   = Migraine
Mth U = Mouth ulcers
TLE   = Temporal lobe epilepsy

their components has the abnormal bowel biopsy that traditionally confirms celiac disease. But if their allergies are severe enough, they are definitely latent celiacs, with all the potential for trouble of full-fledged celiac sufferers. Jill was well and truly in that category. If she didn't have celiac disease, she was certainly right on the verge of it.

That made me wonder about young Craig. Did Jill's condition suggest anything about his likely problem? It did – his tests revealed marked allergies to wheat and legumes. He didn't yet have celiac disease, but he was well on the way.

Interesting . . . although, on its own, inconclusive.

However, it didn't stay on its own for long. Within a fairly short time I had seen a number of Down's Syndrome children, collected their family trees, and been struck by the similarity of the patterns emerging.

THE JENKINS FAMILY: CONTINUING THE PATTERN

A typical one is provided by the Jenkins family (*Figure 31*). Little Karen Jenkins, a six-year-old with Down's Syndrome child, is the youngest of 10 children. I still recall the day that her mother Grace brought her in. As soon as I started talking to Grace, I couldn't help thinking, "Here we go again."

Before a single test was done, I suspected that Grace, then 43, would have autoimmune disease. I could see straight away that she had white dots in her fingernails and vitiligo (patches of white skin). Both are often the result of vitamin and mineral malabsorption caused by food allergies – a condition that goes right along with autoimmune disease.

Tests soon showed that Grace did indeed have a whole range of autoimmune antibodies. And when I saw her family tree, I wasn't surprised. Her father, as you can see, had cancer of the pancreas, with vitiligo thrown in. One aunt also had cancer of the pancreas. Another had thyroid disorder. And the last one had diabetes. When you

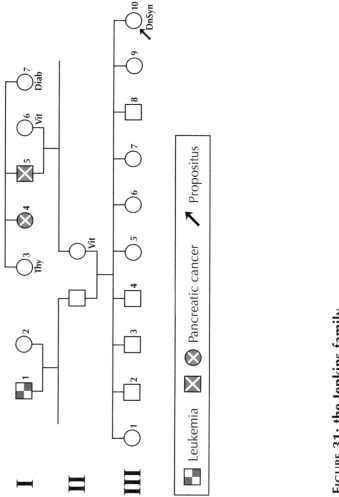

FIGURE 31: the Jenkins family

The Down's Syndrome/celiac-disease link continues.

Diab	= Diabetes	Thy	= Thyroid disorder
Dn Syn	= Down's syndrome	Vit	= Vitiligo

see a family like that, celiac disease is the first thing you think of. While Grace probably didn't have celiac disease in the true sense, she most definitely had its first cousin.

No such doubt existed, however, with young Karen. Her pathology tests showed the classic pattern of celiac disease. And one other thing on the family tree caught my eye – her paternal grandfather had died of leukemia.

THE PATERSON FAMILY: THE PATTERN SWITCHES SIDES

An intriguing twist on the emerging patterns came with the Paterson family. Most of my Down's Syndrome family trees do show definite indications of celiac disease in the mother's family: but take a look at the Paterson family tree (*Figure 32*).

Little Kelvin Paterson, a Down's Syndrome child, was only seven months old. For various reasons, we couldn't get his mother Gail's family tree – although her phenotype of a pale, freckled face and ginger hair is one that goes with an above-average incidence of grain allergies.

However, Kelvin's father, Ken, offered to compile his family tree. I wasn't sure whether that would mean a lot, but I told him to go ahead.

When I saw it, I was very glad I did.

Ken himself had the fissured tongue that results from Vitamin B_3 deficiency. His mother had died of melanoma, the deadly black mole skin cancer – one in twelve of which is hereditary, or due to hereditary factors (see Chapter 7). Ken's father had arthritis. One of his uncles had bowel cancer, the other had throat cancer, and his aunt had leukemia. His paternal grandmother had stomach cancer and arthritis.

A picture more suggestive of a celiac-disease family would be hard to imagine. But here it was occurring on the father's side, not the mother's. Could Ken's apparent celiac family picture have any connection with Kelvin's Down's Syndrome – especially as Gail, at 29, was unusually young for a Down's Syndrome mother?

I believe it could, and I'll explain why in a moment.

Meanwhile, I ran pathology tests on Kelvin and the results were quite definite. Although he was only seven months old, Kelvin's pathology was that of a very severe case of celiac disease.

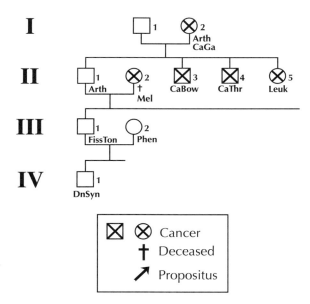

FIGURE 32: the Paterson family

Another celiac-disease picture preceding Down's Syndrome – this time, however, on the father's side.

Arth	= Arthritis
Ca Bow	= Bowel cancer
Ca Ga	= Gastric (stomach) cancer
Ca Thr	= Throat cancer
Dn Syn	= Down's syndrome
Fiss Ton	= Fissured tongue (? low B_3)
Leuk	= Leukemia
Mel	= Melanoma
Phen	= Phenotype – pale, freckled face, ginger hair – (associated with higher incidence of grain allergies, celiac disease)

Because of the message of these and other family trees, I started to wonder. Down's Syndrome children are short for their age, are very prone to infections, have learning difficulties, poor coordination and a high risk for cancer, leukemia and psychiatric disorders.

For decades, everyone has assumed that those things stem from the chromosomal abnormality that underlies the whole syndrome. And yet, they're precisely the problems that other children with celiac disease tend to have.

FROM CHROMOSOMES – OR CELIAC DISEASE?

Could it be that those problems in Down's Syndrome children come, not so much from the chromosomal abnormalities, but from celiac disease?

It was a revolutionary idea. And yet, the family trees that I was amassing seemed to be propelling me in that direction. So I resolved to do something that, as far as I know, no one else has ever done on a regular basis. I decided to run pathology tests associated with celiac disease on every Down's Syndrome child who came in my door.

The outcome, to say the least, has been staggering. I have to date tested 18 Down's syndrome children – and 17 of them have the pathology associated with celiac disease. The one exception was Craig Hopkins, who, as we've seen, was well on his way to developing it. The implications of this are quite breathtaking. By being placed on a gluten-free diet with the right amounts of relevant vitamins and minerals, most of those 18 children have made rapid and measurable improvements in height, head circumference, weight, mental and motor development and general health.

What does that mean for the thousands of Down's Syndrome children throughout the world – almost all of whom are just not being tested for celiac disease, auto-immune disease, food allergies and vitamin-mineral deficiencies?

ALZHEIMER'S DISEASE: SOME NEW INSIGHTS?

While we're pondering that, let's consider something else. Down's Syndrome children have another noticeable characteristic – a very high percentage of them develop Alzheimer's disease around the age of 35 to 40.

Why do they do so? Once again, it has always been assumed that the chromosomal abnormality is somehow to blame. But now, after observing celiac disease indications or their beginnings in 18 out of 18 Down's Syndrome children, I'm starting to see another possibility. Celiac disease stems from grain allergies – or, more precisely, allergies to the gluten and α-gliadin components of grain. As we saw in Chapter 8, those allergies cause malabsorption, and hence a massive deficiency of Vitamins B_1, B_3, B_{12} and folic acid, and the mineral zinc. A serious deficiency in any one of those, if undiagnosed or untreated, can cause dementia.

The allergies also cause malabsorption of essential minerals and trace elements such as calcium, magnesium, iron and manganese. In addition, they allow the absorption of toxic metals such as aluminum and higher than normal concentrations of aluminum in the brain is one of the dementia-causing features of Alzheimer's disease.

Finally, gluten/α-gliadin sensitivity not only lowers vitamin-mineral absorption, but also is directly toxic in its own right. It has been observed to cause degeneration of the central nervous system, and so can actually be a prime cause of dementia on its own.

So, if celiac disease and its accompanying gluten/α-gliadin sensitivity can do all that, and if it's so common in Down's Syndrome children, isn't it possible that it, and not the chromosomal abnormality, is the main reason so many of these children go on to develop Alzheimer's disease?

I'm sure it is.

TWO EXCITING POSSIBILITIES

If I'm right, two more exciting consequences follow.

First, something can now be done to protect Down's Syndrome people from Alzheimer's disease in adult life. And second, we have a very important clue to the cause of Alzheimer's disease itself. For if unsuspected celiac disease causes it in Down's Syndrome people, mightn't it do so in other folks as well? Just think of the prospects for prevention, and even cures, if the answer turns out to be "yes." In Chapter 8, we saw that Alzheimer's disease frequently appears in an autosomal dominant pattern, although some researchers think that a slow virus of some kind could be involved too. We also noted that no one yet knows how to treat it or prevent it.

If my theory is right, we now know how to do both. And we can see why the disease often seems to be autosomal dominant. What is actually being transmitted is a hereditary sensitivity to gluten and α-gliadin, which could also make people susceptible to a slow-acting virus, if indeed one is involved.

This would mean that Alzheimer's disease is actually one of the grain-allergy-based dementias that we discussed early in Chapter 8, rather than the purely genetic and/or viral disease it is now assumed to be.

I would love to see lots of family trees of people who have been diagnosed as having Alzheimer's disease, and scan them for grain-allergy signs – unfortunately, I don't have many in my files. That's because virtually all the dementias I have seen have either fallen into the grain allergy category, or have been due to undiagnosed SLE.

I do, however, have one small family tree that includes a man diagnosed as having Alzheimer's disease. He had been dead for some time, but I saw his son, who had the symptoms of paranoid schizophrenia, plus the very definite grain-allergy signs of celiac disease and gluten sensitivity. But attractive though they are, these theories about celiac disease and grain allergies being the common link between Down's Syndrome, Alzheimer's disease, lymphoma and leukemia are still only theories. What we need now are a lot more family trees, to see if the celiac-disease/grain-allergy/α-gliadin and gluten-sensitivity picture remains constant – and if it does, a lot of research to confirm its truth.

Family trees on their own, let me emphasize, can never be the final proof of any of these theories, but what they can do is to point researchers in the right direction . . . and so save years of time, zillions of dollars in research costs, and a great deal of human suffering.

A LEAP OF INTUITION

Putting it another way, family trees are a launching pad for a leap of intuition. And the leap of intuition I've taken from my Down's Syndrome family trees hasn't yet brought me back to earth.

I've already mentioned how I believe grain allergies cause the dementia symptoms of Alzheimer's disease. And in Chapter 7, I outlined my theory of how they cause cancer. Now, from where I am in mid-leap, so to speak, I think I can just see how they might cause Down's Syndrome and its associated high risk for leukemia.

Please follow me while I complete my leap – because, let me repeat, if I'm right the possibilities for good are very extensive indeed.

You'll remember that celiac disease's accompanying grain allergy (or gluten sensitivity) drastically lowers your body's absorption of several vital substances. These include Vitamins B_1 and B_3, zinc, calcium, magnesium and manganese. They also include Vitamins C and B_6. Consequently, if you have celiac disease, you'll also have markedly low levels of most of those vitamins and minerals, and this can have consequences quite beyond the ones we've already considered.

A low enough level of Vitamin B_1, for instance, will interfere with the body's production of a chemical called cyclic adenosine monophosphate – or cAMP, for short.

At the same time, severely reduced levels of Vitamins C, B_3 and B_6, along with zinc, magnesium and manganese can result in underproduction of prostaglandins of the E1 Series and overproduction of prostaglandins of the E2 Series – commonly abbreviated to PGE2.

Now, just the right balance of cAMP and PGE2 is needed for normal cell division (meiosis). Consequently, I believe that the imbalance of cAMP and PGE2 caused by celiac disease in the mother, or possibly even the father, could well cause the abnormal cell division of Down's Syndrome – which, you'll remember, is characterized by 47 chromosomes in every cell, instead of 46. The imbalance could also cause the condition found in some children who don't have Down's Syndrome, but who do have 47 chromosomes instead of 46 in the bone marrow cells. And it's their faulty bone marrow that puts these children and Down's Syndrome children so much at risk for leukemia.

Going off at a slight tangent, the theory has some interesting implications for cancer research. If the imbalance does indeed cause the abnormal chromosomal changes of Down's Syndrome, could it also be the reason for precancerous chromosomal changes in vulnerable bowel- and breast-tissue cells?

Well, I've landed from my leap of intuition. Let's now think about the consequences, if my leap turns out to be on target.

DOWN'S SYNDROME: NEW HOPE FOR TREATMENT . . . AND PREVENTION?

If I'm right, all Down's Syndrome children should totally avoid gluten, α-gliadin and other toxic fractions of grains – meaning, of course, a grain-free diet. They should also be supplemented with the relevant vitamins and minerals that their bodies have not been able to absorb.

From my experience, remarkable, and measurable, improvements in their intelligence, height and general health will quickly follow. Their chances of getting Alzheimer's disease in adulthood will, if I'm right, be almost zero. Even their risks for bowel cancer, leukemia and thyroid disorder will be enormously reduced.

There are many other exciting possibilities for prevention, too. Every mother-to-be with a family tree suggestive of celiac disease, grain allergies, gluten sensitivity or autoimmune disease should have her allergies identified, avoid the offending foods and take vitamin-mineral supplements during pregnancy. This especially applies to older mothers, whose egg cells are more likely to be below par anyway. It could well apply to men with that sort of family tree: If the imbalance does affect the meiosis of male reproductive cells, avoiding suspect foods and taking vitamin-mineral supplements for as long as possible before conception would obviously be valuable. And the vitamin-mineral supplements would be an excellent idea for women who have had prepregnancy abdominal x-rays, which can be another cause of low Vitamin B_1 and PGE1 series.

If those steps are taken, and my theory is right, far fewer children will be born with Down's Syndrome. And even that's not all. If Alzheimer's disease is indeed a grain-allergy-based condition, the disease and all its misery can be virtually eliminated by diet and a few vitamin-mineral supplements.

Just imagine the benefits for humanity implied in the last few paragraphs. What a field for research – and what a potential for the relief of suffering! I believe that's the kind of hope that can come from the study of family trees.

For some people I've seen who had cancer, or were at extreme risk for it, that hope has come already.

FAMILY TREES THAT CONQUERED CANCER

In Chapter 7, I outlined my theories as to how cancer can be caused by hereditary food allergies and autoimmune disease – conditions that usually stand out clearly in a family tree. I also promised to provide some family trees that would not only support the theory, but also illustrate the possibilities for prevention, treatment, and even cures that flow from it.

Now, here they are. To start them off, let's consider the thought-provoking case of Cathy.

Cathy: Her depression was only the beginning

It was her depression that first brought Cathy to see me. And considering what was wrong with her, it was no wonder she was depressed.

Five months previously, cancer had been diagnosed in her left breast and the nodes in her armpit. She had been advised to have the breast removed, but had refused. Nor was she prepared to have the chemotherapy and ray treatment that her doctors had recommended.

In addition, she had chronic anxiety, tiredness, chronic loose bowel motions, arthritis and a history of alcoholism. To complete the picture, her hair was falling out.

Clearly, treating her depression while ignoring her cancer would have been a classic case of rearranging the deck chairs on the Titanic. But already I was wondering if the two weren't somehow related.

And when I saw her family tree (*Figure 33*), I was sure of it.

Cathy wasn't the first in her family to have breast cancer. Her aunt Enid had also been a victim. Her cousin Peter had died of cancer at 32. And her grandfather Ben had died of Hodgkin's disease (cancer of the lymph system) at 48.

Four cancers in three generations. Now, cast your mind back again to Chapter 7. You'll recall my claim that, whenever a family has an unusually high incidence of cancer, you almost always find evidence of autoimmune disease accompanying it. And there it was in Cathy's family – in aunt Enid's thyroid disorder (which led to her thyroid gland being removed) and the arthritis suffered by Cathy's other aunt, Flora.

As soon as I saw those conditions plus the other cancers, I was sure that here we had a family with hereditary autoimmune disease, probably caused by grain allergies, coming from grandfather Ben in an X-linked dominant pattern. In which case, Cathy was very likely to have autoimmune disease, with severe allergies to grains and perhaps a few other things, like milk, lying behind it.

Then I glanced at the other side of Cathy's family. Not much there – except that Cathy's father Joe had shared her alcoholism, and her paternal grandfather Claude had suffered from quite serious depression. Alcoholism is often associated with yeast, malt and grain allergies. And depression, as we've seen several times, frequently comes from grain allergies. If it had done so in Claude's case, Cathy may well have received grain-allergy tendencies from both sides.

Two questions remained. Did Cathy really have autoimmune disease and grain and milk allergies, and maybe (considering the alcoholism) yeast allergies too? If so – and this was the big question – were those things indeed causing the cancer in her and her relatives?

The first question was easily answered. Tests showed that she did have the pathology of autoimmune disease, plus milk, grain, eggs and beef allergies and vitamin/mineral deficiencies. The yeast allergies were somewhat borderline, but the whole picture pointed to celiac disease in no uncertain manner.

The second question was rather more difficult to answer. In fact, the only way of answering it was to put her on a strict diet that avoided her allergies, give her plenty of the vitamins and minerals that she was malabsorbing, and see what happened.

Cathy cooperated wholeheartedly. She kept rigidly to the diet and regularly took her vitamins and minerals.

And her cancer went away: or, to use the medical term, it *went into remission*.

That was two years ago. There has been no sign of the cancer recurring. Her depression, anxiety and other odds and ends have improved immeasurably. In fact, her only problem has been a bout of hepatitis – the fact that she recovered quickly was itself a pointer to her improved heath and revitalized immune system.

So the answer to the second question also appears to be "yes." The fact that she got better when it was treated indicates that the autoimmune disease, with its underlying allergies and vitamin-mineral deficiencies, was indeed causing Cathy's cancer. As it seems to have been

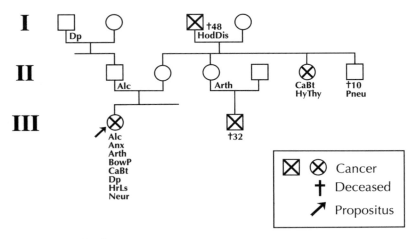

FIGURE 33: Cathy

Four cancers, plus evidence of autoimmune disease and grain allergies. When we treated Cathy's grain allergies and consequent vitamin-mineral deficiencies, her cancer cleared up.

Alc	= Alcoholism
Anx	= Chronic anxiety
Arth	= Arthritis
Bow P	= Chronic loose bowel motions
Ca Bt	= Breast cancer with secondary cancer in armpit
Dp	= Depression
Hod Dis	= Hodgkin's disease
Hr Ls	= Hair loss
Hy Thy	= Hyperthyroidism with thyroidectomy (removal of thyroid gland)
Neur	= Neurasthenia (chronic lack of energy)
Pneu	= Pneumonia

running in her family for some time, it's logical to assume that it also caused her relatives' cancers.

This means that the progression of cancer through Cathy's family can now be stopped because the family tree revealed that it has an identifiable, and readily treatable, cause.

How many other families does that apply to – but who have never had their family trees studied, and the relevant tests done?

ROBYN: A RAPIDLY GROWING CANCER

It certainly applied to Robyn, who came to see me in a state of great fear and depression.

She had had bowel cancer for some time, and had been advised to try a vegetarian diet. There did seem to be some improvement at first, but now the cancer was really making a comeback. An ultrascan test showed that it was growing rapidly.

Not a happy situation. But not a mysterious one, either, once her family tree (*Figure 34*) had been compiled.

Just have a look at it. Robyn's father Don and her paternal uncle and aunt all had dementia. Her mother Jill had depressive illness and Parkinson's disease. Jill's two brothers had bowel cancer and stomach cancer – and both their parents had had mood swings and depression.

Robyn's paternal grandfather Harold died of esophageal cancer. Her paternal grandmother Myrtle suffered kidney failure. Back in the present generations, Robyn's sister Rosalie had asthma, while Rosalie's three boys had asthma, depression and one case of ITP, or low blood-platelet count.

That's not the sort of picture that life insurance salesmen like to see. But it's certainly a revealing one – and I'm sure that, by now, you hardly need me to tell you what it reveals.

If you said "grain allergies," you've been paying attention all through the book.

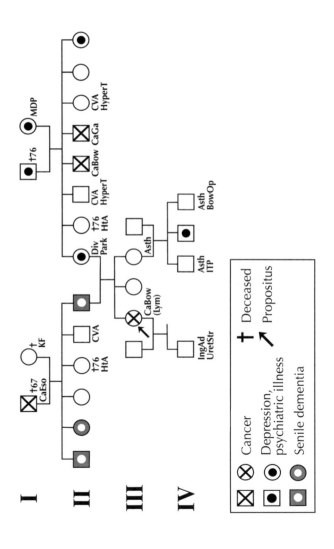

FIGURE 34: Robyn

A clear picture of grain-allergies wreaking havoc on both sides of the family. Robyn's cancer cleared up when her grain-allergy/autoimmune-disease picture was corrected.

Asth	= Asthma	Hyper T	= Hypertension
Bow Op	= Bowel operation – intussusception	Ing Ad	= Inguinal adenitis (swollen groin glands)
Ca Bow (Lym)	= Bowel cancer – lymphoma	ITP	= Low blood platelet count
Ca Ga	= Gastric (stomach) cancer	KF	= Kidney failure
Ca Eso	= Cancer of esophagus	MDP	= Manic-depressive illness
CVA	= Cardiovascular accident (stroke)	Park Dis	= Parkinson's disease
Div	= Diverticulitis	Uret Str	= Blocked urethra
Ht A	= Heart attack		

Rarely, in fact, have I seen a more classic grain-allergy pattern. Running tests on Robyn was almost a formality. But run them I did, and the results were precisely what I expected. Hefty allergies to whole wheat, gluten, eggs, yeast, beef, pork and milk, plus the usual associated vitamin-mineral deficiencies. And, of course, autoimmune disease thrown in.

The irony was that Robyn's vegetarian diet included heaps of molasses, yogurt, bread rolls and wheat bran. So while it successfully got her off beef and pork, it replaced them with plenty of other things at least as damaging, if not more so. However, that damage could now, I hoped, be reversed. The next step was a strict allergy-free diet for Robyn, backed up with relevant vitamins and minerals. And the result?

Her cancer went into remission. Subsequent ultrascan tests showed that it was shrinking as rapidly as it had grown. Once again, we had the same picture – cancer in an autoimmune-disease/grain-allergy family, showing dramatic improvement once those hereditary conditions were corrected.

You can see why I claimed, in Chapter 7, that every cancer patient should be tested for the presence of autoimmune antibodies to the subfractions of grains, eggs, beef and yeast – especially if there are food-allergy signs in the family tree.

CHARMAINE: A SAD IRONY

Thanks to her family tree, Robyn is alive and well today, two years after she came to see me. That can't, unfortunately, be said about Charmaine; and yet Charmaine's story provides extra evidence for the truth of my family-tree-inspired theories.

There was only one word for Charmaine's condition when I first saw her: hopeless. She had already lost her right breast to cancer. Now she had a massive cancer the size of an orange in her left breast. What was more, the cancer on the right-hand side had recurred and grown right through the rib cage, leaving a constantly weeping wound.

The best efforts of a stream of physicians, cancer specialists, radiologists and surgeons had been of no avail. Radiation therapy, surgery, and medication had all failed to halt Charmaine's cancer. Her life expectancy could be measured in weeks: maybe two months at the most.

With a distinct sense of merely going through the motions, I asked her for a family tree. And for once, I didn't feel much better when I saw it (*Figure 35*).

The only things of any consequence on it were breast cancer in Charmaine's maternal grandmother, gall bladder trouble in her mother, TB in her aunt and kidney failure in her cousin. My first reaction was to share the

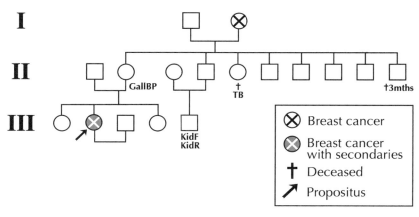

FIGURE 35: Charmaine

A rather sparse family tree: but its pointers to grain allergies provided the key to treating Charmaine's cancer.

Gall B P	= Gall bladder problems
Kid F	= Kidney failure
Kid R	= Both kidneys removed
T B	= Tuberculosis

despair of Charmaine's other doctors. Then I stopped . . .
and did two things.

First, I remembered my own advice: "All cancer
patients should be tested for the presence of autoimmune
antibodies to the subfractions of grains, eggs, beef and
yeast." Then I took another look at the family tree. Breast
cancer, after all, can be associated with grain allergies.
Gall bladder problems do frequently go along with milk,
egg and grain allergies. TB indicates a suppressed immune
system, which is certainly a pointer to food allergies.
And, while kidney failure is by no means always linked
with food allergies, sometimes it is.

Some may have said it was too late to bother, but I
decided to give food allergies a try. Anyway, what did
Charmaine have to lose? Nothing at all. And as it turned
out, she had an enormous amount to gain.

Charmaine proved to be massively allergic to twelve
foods, including grains, legumes and yeast. She was malabsorbing vitamins and minerals as though they didn't
exist, and to judge by her low lymphocyte count, her
immune system had virtually packed up and retired. It
was somewhat past the eleventh hour; nevertheless, I put
her on the appropriate and very tough diet, and pumped
her full of the relevant vitamins and minerals.

Even so, I wasn't really prepared for what happened
. . . the massive breast cancer cleared up . . . the chest
wall healed. Despite their advanced nature, Charmaine's
cancers went into total remission.

The long shot had paid off. Slender as they were, the
family tree's clues had pointed in the right direction. In
Charmaine's case, the cancers were obviously being
caused by the allergies, vitamin-mineral deficiencies and
autoimmune disease. Clear them up and you cleared up
the cancer. Suddenly, Charmaine's two-month life
expectancy increased to an indefinite future.

But 15 months later the final blow came. After enjoying more than a year of excellent health, Charmaine died
of fibrosis of the lungs – a delayed result of her earlier
radiation therapy.

It was a supreme irony. Because of the treatment suggested by her family tree, Charmaine beat the cancer, only to die from the effects of a previous form of treatment. It wasn't the happy ending that everyone wanted, but it was surely a case of great significance for cancer research.

These are just three case histories that give weight to my theory; namely, that when cancer occurs frequently in families, the most likely cause is hereditary autoimmune disease, especially celiac disease and SLE. If my theory is true, perhaps the most exciting aspect of it is the opportunities it creates for cancer prediction and prevention.

Let's look at two case histories that not only buttress the theory further, but also are examples, I believe, of the prevention of cancers that would otherwise almost certainly have developed.

SARAH: A WELL-FOUNDED FEAR OF CANCER

Sarah was very worried indeed when she came into my surgery. Depression and lack of energy were her expressed reasons for coming, but a deeper reason lurked behind them: The fear of cancer.

And in Sarah's case, the fear was well founded. When you look at her family tree (*Figure 36*), I think you'll agree.

Her mother had died of breast cancer, her uncle of lung cancer, her grandmother of stomach cancer and her great-grandmother of bowel cancer.

With a history like that, there just had to be some hereditary factor at work. And as usual, the autoimmune-disease/allergy indications were there, making no secret of their presence.

They began with the pernicious anemia back in Sarah's grandmother. They continued with the anemia in Sarah's mother Yvonne. They were hinted at in the colitis suffered by Yvonne and her brother Martin (colitis is a bowel irritation that frequently has an allergic base, and can be a first step toward bowel cancer).

They surfaced in Sarah's brother, Peter and sister, Tracy, who are twins. Peter, as you can see, has asthma and migraine. He has also had hepatitis, which could indicate immune system suppression. Tracy has migraine, irritable bowel (a first cousin of colitis) and mood swings.

Right down to Sarah's children, the indications continue. Tom has known allergies to chocolate and oranges, and Joan has a milk allergy. Tom also has ITP, the low blood platelet count that we saw previously in Robyn's family. Interestingly enough, both Tom and Joan have pyloric stenosis (narrowing of the opening out of the stomach), but that's probably unconnected with the main problems.

And what about Sarah herself? Known indications of allergies abounded with her, too. She had suffered an attack of what sounded like Osler's Syndrome (see Chapter 6), where the body swells up in an extreme allergic reaction. Oranges, chocolate, wine and cola gave her migraine. She was also known to be allergic to yeast, milk and molds. To add further substance to her cancer fears, five nonmalignant lumps had already been removed from her breasts.

I wasn't surprised at what my further tests revealed. Besides her known problems, Sarah had severe allergies to grains, malt, rice and goat's milk. She was extremely low in Vitamins B_1, B_6, C and E and essential trace elements, despite the fact that she took supplements of them all. She had an autoimmune-disease picture that suggested celiac disease, definite indications of SLE, and, I'm certain, a very high chance of following in her forebears' footsteps and developing cancer.

I'm sure, however, that what is really being transmitted through Sarah's family is not cancer itself but hereditary autoimmune disease, which is causing the cancer. The transmission could be X-linked dominant or autosomal dominant. Either way, Sarah was right in the firing line for it, and copped it in full measure – and with it, an extreme risk for cancer.

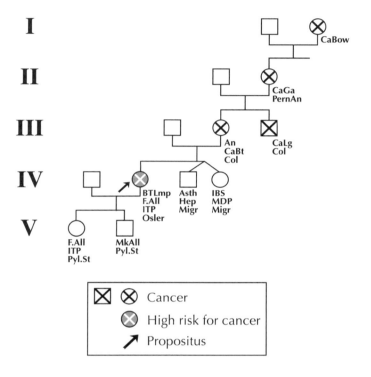

FIGURE 36: Sarah

A string of cancers – once again accompanied by the unmistakable signs of autoimmune disease and food allergies.

An	= Anemia	Hep	= Hepatitis
Asth	= Asthma	I B S	= Irritable bowel syndrome
Bt Lmp	= Breast lump	ITP	= Low blood-platelet count
Ca Bow	= Bowel cancer	MDP	= Manic-depressive illness
Ca Bt	= Breast cancer	Migr	= Migraine
Ca Ga	= Gastric (stomach) cancer	Mk All	= Milk allergies
		Osler	= Osler's syndrome
Ca Lg	= Lung cancer	Pern An	= Pernicious anemia
Col	= Colitis	Pyl St	= Pyloric stenosis
F All	= Food allergies		

In turn, that risk was shared by her brother and sister, and had been transmitted to her children.

Now, however, the risk has been unmasked. With allergy-free diets and relevant vitamins and minerals, Sarah and all her family should not only dodge the cancer completely, but also enjoy much better general health.

Today, more than two years later, Sarah's health has indeed improved immensely. And she shows no signs whatsoever of developing cancer.

Maria: eight cancers in two generations

Awesome though it was, Sarah's family history of cancer was confined to her mother's side. In Maria's family, the cancer was rampant on both sides, making Maria's chances of avoiding it look very slim indeed.

Maria's family (*Figure 37*) was, in fact, one of the most remarkable cancer families I have yet seen. Both her father George and her mother Jean had died of multiple cancers – George of the lungs and stomach, Jean of the cervix (neck of the womb) and ovary. George's mother had died of cancer of the cervix and stomach, and Jean's parents had died of cancer of the bowel and cervix, respectively.

Jean's mother had married twice. Her three sons of the second marriage (Jean's half-brothers) all had cancer – two of the pancreas and one of the lung.

Eight cancers in two generations. An appalling picture indeed – one that amply justified the fear of cancer that had haunted Maria for years, and underlay the depression that brought her to me.

Unfortunately, we couldn't get much information about other conditions that might have existed in Maria's relatives. But I really didn't need more. A cancer history like hers had to have a reason, and once again I was prepared to bet that hereditary autoimmune disease was it.

Strengthening my confidence was the fact that Maria had depression, arthritis and colitis. Her other problems included a 2.7-kg dermoid cyst that she'd had for 40 years. This had recently been found and removed during a hysterectomy. She also had a duodenal ulcer, and pancreatitis which, considering the pancreatic cancer in her two uncles, was possibly precancerous in her case.

The usual tests gave the usual results. Maria was very allergic to grains, malt, cocoa and carrots. Her vitamin-mineral levels were way down. She had autoimmune disease and all the indications of SLE. To me, there was one inescapable conclusion: Maria was the product of two families in which hereditary autoimmune disease was causing cancer – two families that had come together to bequeath her a double dose of autoimmune-disease genes and an overwhelming cancer risk.

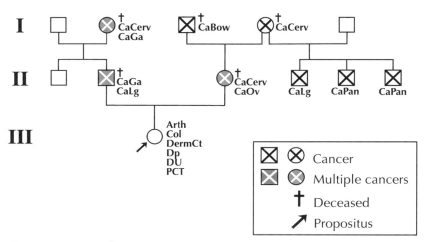

FIGURE 37: Maria
With eight cancers in two generations of her family, Maria's fear of the disease was amply justified.

Arth	= Arthritis	Ca Pan	= Pancreatic cancer
Ca Bow	= Bowel cancer	Col	= Colitis
Ca Cer	= Cervical cancer	Derm Ct	= Dermoid cyst
Ca Ga	= Gastric (stomach) cancer	Dp	= Depression
		DU	= Duodenal ulcer
Ca Lg	= Lung cancer	PCT	= Pancreatitis
Ca Ov	= Ovarian cancer		

But once again, we had got in under the wire. Maria is now doing extremely well on her allergy-free diet and relevant vitamins and minerals. Nearly three years after I first saw her, she is in excellent general health. She remains totally free of cancer; even her pancreatitis has cleared up.

Now, what are we to make of family histories like these last five? I believe they can't be ignored or shrugged off as coincidences. I believe they provide powerful evidence that, in many families, cancer is caused by hereditary autoimmune disease and its associated food allergies.

I believe I have demonstrated that, in such cases, cancer can be prevented – and cured – by heeding the evidence of the family tree and treating the autoimmune disease.

Here, I am certain, is one of the most promising directions yet for cancer research. And – a very exciting thought – it's a research program in which you can become involved . . . simply by drawing up your family tree.

❧13❧

Cures for Incurable Illnesses Through Family Trees?

For all its menace and unresolved mysteries, cancer is a disease that can very often be cured. Let's end the book by looking at three conditions usually regarded as totally incurable – and make a few speculations about them in the light of some fascinating family trees.

The conditions are Duchenne muscular dystrophy, motor neuron disease or amyotrophic lateral sclerosis (ALS for short) and multiple sclerosis. The textbooks say that their causes are unknown, and that no effective treatment is available for any of them.

I wonder . . .

The distinguishing effect of Duchenne muscular dystrophy is that it causes a progressive weakening and wasting away of the muscles. It is known to be inherited, in an X-linked recessive way.

Consequently, it appears almost exclusively in boys, while girls become carriers for it (see Chapter 2 for an explanation of why that happens).

When a mother is a carrier, each son has a 50 percent chance of getting the condition, and each daughter has a 50 percent chance of being a carrier.

The initial symptom is usually a waddling style of walk, because the hip and leg muscles seem to be affected first. The boy finds it hard to climb stairs or to get up from the floor. Soon after, the arms start to grow weaker.

Once the symptoms appear, improvement is virtually unknown. In most cases, sufferers are confined to bed or a wheelchair by the time they are 12. They rarely live much past 20.

THE KENTS: A DIAGNOSIS OF DOOM

Against that background, let's consider the Kent family (*Figure 38*) and their two boys, Neville and Jason.

Their mother brought them to me back in 1979, when Neville was six and Jason was four. The previous year, both had been positively diagnosed as having Duchenne muscular dystrophy. This was done by muscle biopsies, and by measuring their levels of an enzyme called creatine phosphokinase (CPK), which leaks into the blood from damaged muscle tissue. Neville's CPK level was 11,000. Jason's was 8000. When you consider that the normal level is less than 85, you can see the significance of those readings.

If further confirmation of the diagnosis were needed, it came from the fact that, as you can see from the family tree, Duchenne muscular dystrophy had claimed the lives of the boys' two maternal uncles. I mention these points to emphasize that the boys really did have Duchenne muscular dystrophy, and not one of the enzyme or metabolic disturbances that are sometimes mistaken for it.

So there I was, looking at two young boys with an incurable disease, and thinking about all those textbooks that assured me there was nothing I could do. However, there was one germ of an idea stirring in my mind. And in that sort of situation, almost anything is worth a try.

The germ of an idea centered on the fact that Duchenne muscular dystrophy is an X-linked recessive illness. Now, way back in Chapter 3, I stated what I believe is a principle concerning X-linked illnesses. I think they are frequently linked genetically with a treatable X-linked condition, and if you treat the condition, you treat the illness too.

What were the chances, I wondered, of finding a treatable X-linked condition in this family, accompanying the Duchenne muscular dystrophy?

Admittedly there weren't a lot of clues in the family tree. Mrs. Kent had a history of depression and gastric upsets, which were possible pointers to food allergies, but there was no way of knowing if anything else apart from

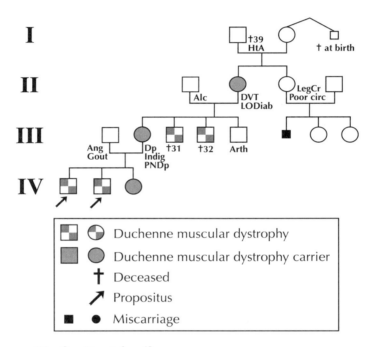

FIGURE 38: the Kent family

Both the Kent boys were victims of Duchenne muscular dystrophy, a devastating, incurable condition that had claimed the lives of their two uncles. So the boys faced certain death by their early 20s – or did they?

Alc	= Alcoholism	Indig	= Indigestion
Ang	= Angina	Leg Cr	= Leg cramps
Arth	= Arthritis	L O Diab	= Late-onset diabetes
Dp	= Depression	M C	= Miscarriage
DVT	= Deep vein thrombosis	P N Dp	= Postnatal depression
Ht A	= Heart attack	Poor Circ	= Poor circulation

muscular dystrophy had affected her long-dead brothers. Little or no information was available on other members of her family.

Mr. Kent's family, of course, wasn't relevant, as the muscular dystrophy was all coming from Mrs. Kent's side. So, if anything were going to be discovered, it would have to be through tests.

Accordingly, I ran pathology tests on Neville, Jason and Mrs. Kent. Something very significant did indeed turn up. Despite the fact that they all took vitamin supplements, all three turned out to be extremely low in vitamins, especially Vitamin E. Quite obviously, something was causing a massive vitamin malabsorption, and the tests pointed accusingly at grain, milk, egg, beef and yeast allergies which, given the nature of the family's problems, were probably X-linked.

Was this, then, the treatable X-linked condition accompanying the X-linked muscular dystrophy? It was worth considering – especially as Vitamin E is known to play an important part in the development and maintenance of healthy muscle tissue.

I acted to correct the boys' vitamin deficiencies. It took a bit of doing, but eventually we raised their vitamin levels to somewhere around normal.

Within eight months, their muscular dystrophy pathology was greatly improved. Their CPK readings had dropped quite considerably. At the same time, there was a marked improvement in their overall condition. Today, four years later, they show no sign of further muscle deterioration, and appear to be growing normally.

Why?

Was it a coincidence, a *spontaneous remission*, a wrong diagnosis in the first place, as some doctors have claimed? Or was it a vindication of my theory that if you treat a curable X-linked condition that's accompanying an X-linked illness, you treat the illness too? And if so, what does it tell us about the real nature of Duchenne muscular dystrophy? What is really being transmitted through these unfortunate families? Does this case point to hope, where none existed before?

These questions arise irresistibly from the Kent family's experience. And no researcher working on Duchenne muscular dystrophy can, I believe, afford to ignore them.

As of now, however, the official medical position is that the outlook for anyone with Duchenne muscular dystrophy is black indeed. And for people with motor neuron disease, or ALS, most doctors' forecasts would be even grimmer – three years of life, at the most, from the time of diagnosis.

THE TRAGEDY OF ALS

ALS, as we'll call it for simplicity's sake, is a terrible disease indeed. A neuro-muscular illness, it causes a gradual paralysis of the muscles that eventually leaves the victim totally helpless and bedridden. Death usually comes through an inability to breathe or swallow, or through an infection like pneumonia, which develops more readily when a person is totally inactive.

About the only good thing about ALS is that it's fairly rare. Most doctors would only see three or four cases in their working lives, but the suffering incurred by those few patients is hard to forget.

The first ALS sufferer I saw was Henry, a 70-year-old man who had already beaten the odds by surviving for seven years after his ALS had been diagnosed. Interestingly enough, he had been on a gluten-free diet all that time. He had walked until 18 months before I saw him, but was now confined to a wheelchair.

As a young man, Henry had drunk large amounts of milk. That was significant, because some studies have shown a link between high milk intake and ALS. Later on, he lived in a wheat-growing area and ate lots of wheat; during that time his hair fell out and he developed vitiligo (white patches of skin). Milk and grain allergies leapt into my mind while Henry was still recounting his story. And it was interesting that his mother had had osteoarthritis, a condition that is definitely associated with gluten and gliadin sensitivity, and has an immunology quite similar to that of celiac disease.

On the basis of those observations, I tested Henry for grain and milk allergies. He had both to a marked degree, with vitamin/mineral deficiencies thrown in. I put him on the appropriate diet and vitamin/mineral supplements.

For the last two years, his condition has not deteriorated any further. In other words, he has survived for nine years since his ALS was first diagnosed, as opposed to the normal three or four years.

Keep Henry's case in mind for a moment – especially those milk allergies . . .

THE MCMASTER FAMILY: AND A LEADING QUESTION

It was somewhat later on that Janice McMaster came to see me, with four young men in tow. Her husband Alf had recently fallen victim to ALS, and he was by no means, she added, the first in his family to do so.

What were the chances of her four sons following suit – and what could be done to prevent it?

I scratched my head and looked out the window. It was a lovely day, and for a moment I wished I were somewhere far away from the surgery and far removed from such leading questions. Then I looked back at this very anxious mother who wasn't prepared to accept medicine's assertion that nothing could be done to prevent or cure ALS.

Suddenly I decided that I wasn't, either. So I asked her for a family tree.

And felt a shock of disbelief when I actually saw it (*Figure 39*). Janice hadn't been kidding when she spoke of other ALS cases in her husband's family. Just count them – no fewer than 12 cases in three generations. You can't tell me that coincidence can produce a pattern like that.

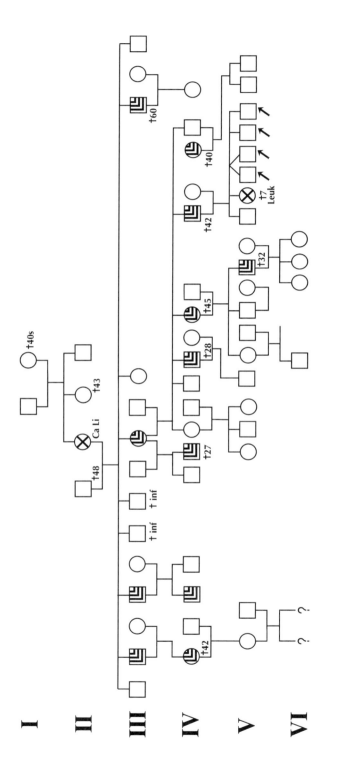

FIGURE 39: the McMaster family

Eleven cases of ALS in three generations: something more than coincidence had to be causing that.

Ca Li = Cancer of liver   Leuk = Leukemia   inf = infancy

Something had to be running through the McMaster family to leave such a trail of devastation.

The questions was – what?

As frequently happens, Janice couldn't get much other medical information, apart from the ALS, into the family tree. So there weren't any hints to be had from that source. But whatever the something was, it was autosomal dominant (not X-linked dominant – see the son-to-son transmission from generations three to four), which meant the four boys were very much at risk.

I ran a full series of tests on all four – and was soon very glad I had done so. All four boys had autoimmune disease and gluten/gliadin allergies. Three of them also had severe milk allergies. The fourth one probably did too, but as he'd been on a milk-free diet for some time, no reaction showed up. In addition, they all had low Vitamin B_6, three had low Vitamin B_1 and two had low Vitamin B_3. Another really significant thing, which I had never expected for a moment, was uncovered.

Each of the four boys had a high level of kryptopyrroles in the urine. By definition, they were all pyrolurics. Now, that really opened up a can of worms. As far as I'm aware, no one else has ever tested potential ALS victims for that kind of thing. Immediately, a host of mind-boggling possibilities arose – and touched off a string of questions.

As we saw in Chapter 10, pyroluria drains the body of Vitamin B_6 and zinc. And Vitamins B_6, B_1 and B_3 aren't absorbed properly if milk allergies are present. So a combination of pyroluria and milk allergies would lead to very low levels of Vitamins B_6 and B_3 indeed. But severely low levels of Vitamins B_6 and B_3 can produce ALS-like symptoms on their own. In fact, symptoms have been deliberately induced in laboratory animals by depriving them of Vitamin B_6.

In the McMaster family, then, are low Vitamins B_6 and B_3 a sign that the boys are indeed heading for ALS? And as milk allergies lead to Vitamin B_6 and B_3 malabsorption, is that why high milk intake and ALS seem to be linked?

For that matter, why do so many ALS sufferers drink a lot of milk? I believe their bodies actually crave it, because it's rich in a substance called tryptophan, the presence of which helps to raise Vitamin B_3 levels. Unfortunately, however, they can't break the tryptophan free from the milk to absorb it because, I believe, their bodies lack certain digestive enzymes. This is another factor in lowering their Vitamin B_3 levels – and their low tryptophan is something else that can cause ALS-like symptoms on its own.

What's more, pyroluria is known to produce neurological symptoms by itself. Does it team up with Vitamins B_6, B_3 and tryptophan deficiencies to produce ALS symptoms in some people?

Then again, pyroluria is often the precursor of porphyria, which is identified by porphyrins as well as kryptopyrroles in the urine. You'll recall that porphyria certainly produces neurological symptoms such as a shuffling gait, foot drop and bulbar palsy (inability to swallow and talk) – symptoms, in fact, that are very like some of the manifestations of ALS.

Will the McMaster boys' pyroluria develop into porphyria? That's something we have to watch over the next few years – especially as porphyria is autosomal dominant, which would fit the ALS pattern in this family precisely.

Which leads me to the two big questions. Have we found, in this family, a hereditary pyroluria with low Vitamins B_6 and B_3 and tryptophan – a combination that, in three generations, has caused 12 cases of an illness indistinguishable from ALS? And taking that question to its logical conclusion: Is ALS really a separate illness, or is it simply a variant of pyroluria and porphyria, with very low levels of Vitamins B_6, B_1 and B_3 and tryptophan?

If so, the consequences would be revolutionary. An unavoidable disease would suddenly become avoidable: easy to predict, easy to prevent. And in those who already had it, further deterioration could be halted.

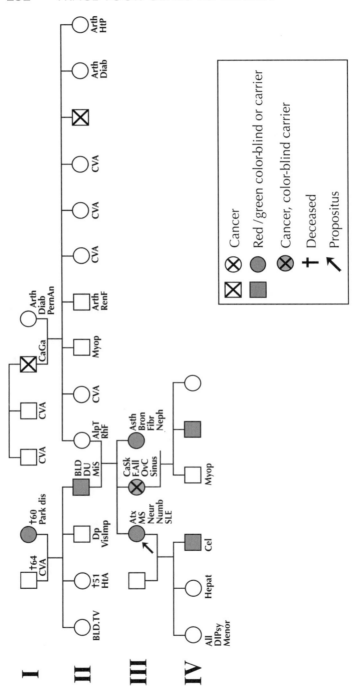

FIGURES 40: Amy, Yvette and Lynne

Three victims of MS – with a remarkably similar pattern in each family tree.

All	= Allergies
Alop Tot	= Total alopecia
Arth	= Arthritis
Atx	= Ataxia
Bld Eye	= Blind in one eye
Bld Tun Vis	= Blind, tunnel vision
Bron	= Bronchitis
Ca Ga	= Gastric (stomach) cancer
Ca Sk	= Skin cancer
Coel Dis	= Celiac disease
CVA	= Cardiovascular accident (stroke)
Dg Ind Psy	= Drug-induced psychosis
Diab	= Diabetes
Dp	= Depression
Duo U	= Duodenal ulcer
Fd All	= Food allergies
Fibr	= Fibrous tumor in womb
Hepat	= Hepatitis
Ht A	= Heart attack
Ht P	= Heart problems
Menor	= Menorrhagia
MS	= Multiple sclerosis
Myop	= Myopathy (muscle disease)
Neph	= Nephritis
Neur	= Neurasthenia
Numb	= Numb left forearm and hands
Ov Cyst	= Ovarian cyst
Park Dis	= Parkinson's disease
Pern An	= Pernicious anemia
Ren F	= Renal failure
Rheum F	= Rheumatic fever
Sinus	= Sinusitis
SLE	= Systemic lupus erythematosus
Vis Imp	= Impaired vision

On the basis of this family tree, can researchers afford to ignore the possibility? With appropriate treatment, the McMaster boys should now avoid developing ALS symptoms. How many other potential victims could avoid them, too, through this approach?

The more family trees I see, the more exciting – and unexpected – are the possibilities they open up. And that's most definitely the case with these last three. They just might shed a ray of hope on one of the most baffling and tragic diseases of all – multiple sclerosis.

A BREAKTHROUGH ON MS – THROUGH FAMILY TREES?

This better known, but equally unpleasant, cousin of ALS attacks the myelin, the sheath around the nerves, and causes a progressive deterioration of the central nervous system and spinal cord. It produces a variety of symptoms, depending on where it strikes, including eyesight and speech problems. Generally, MS robs people of the use of their limbs, confines them to wheelchairs, frequently paralyzes them, and eventually kills them.

Like muscular dystrophy and ALS, MS is regarded as an incurable disease. An enormous amount of research is being poured into it, without concrete results to date. Many researchers are in hot pursuit of a hypothetical virus, and are convinced that the viral trail will eventually lead them to the answer. Well, maybe so. But if the cases of Amy, Yvette and Lynne are any guide, the answer may lie in a totally different direction.

A COMMON PATTERN

Their family trees are *Figures 40, 41* and *42*, respectively. I've grouped them together because, while each has distinctive features, a remarkably similar pattern shows through them all.

Pernicious anemia and mood swings occur in each. Stomach cancer, heart attacks, asthma and Down's

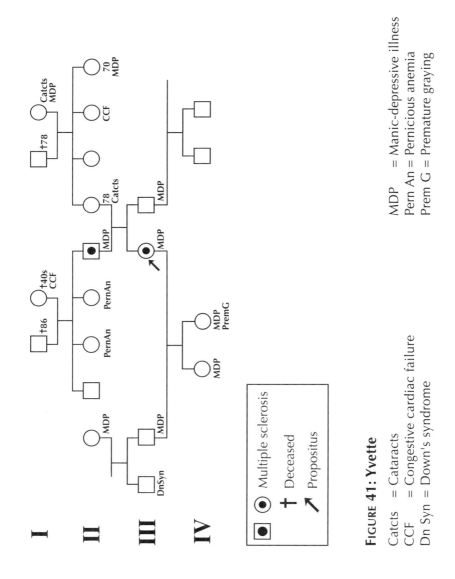

FIGURE 41: Yvette

Catcts = Cataracts
CCF = Congestive cardiac failure
Dn Syn = Down's syndrome

MDP = Manic-depressive illness
Pern An = Pernicious anemia
Prem G = Premature graying

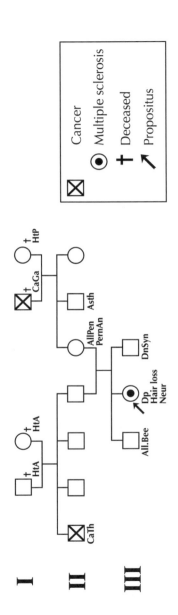

FIGURE 42 : Lynne

All Bee	=	Allergy to bee venom
Asth	=	Asthma
Ca Ga	=	Gastric (stomach) cancer
Ca Th	=	Throat cancer
Dn Syn	=	Down's syndrome
Dp	=	Depression

Ht A	=	Heart attack (coronary occlusion)
Ht P	=	Heart problems
Neur	=	Neurasthenia (chronic lack of energy)
Pen All	=	Penicillin allergy
Pern An	=	Pernicious anemia

Syndrome show up in two. Arthritis and diabetes appear in Amy's extensive family tree. We've met all those conditions a number of times before. What does it mean when they all occur together?

That's right. A family full of hereditary food allergies, leading to vitamin-mineral deficiencies, autoimmune disease and SLE.

In Amy's family, they're probably X-linked. You can see how several of the symptoms are following the red-green color blindness, which is certainly an X-linked condition. And notice in Yvette's family that both she and her father have MS, plus the mood swings that so often accompany hereditary food allergies and their consequences.

Interesting, too, is the presence of Down's Syndrome – although in Yvette's family it is, admittedly, unconnected with her. In the previous chapter we looked at evidence that links Down's Syndrome with grain allergies and celiac disease.

With family backgrounds like those, you can imagine the tests I ran on Amy, Yvette and Lynne. And the results were precisely what you would have expected.

All three ladies had autoimmune disease, food allergies and vitamin-mineral deficiencies. Lynne went one step further and added SLE to the list.

So we have three out of three MS sufferers with autoimmune disease, food allergies and vitamin-mineral deficiencies – and all coming from families exhibiting the autoimmune-disease/SLE syndrome to a marked degree.

SOME FASCINATING IMPLICATIONS

The implications of these results are fascinating. To start with, grain allergies, celiac disease and low Vitamin B_{12} and folate can all cause cerebellar atrophy, a wasting away of the brain tissue – and cerebellar atrophy produces many of the typical MS symptoms.

Low Vitamin B_{12}, another part of the autoimmune-disease pattern, can cause degeneration of the spinal cord, which also produces symptoms just like those of MS.

SLE can cause a condition called transverse myelitis. This is a blockage of small blood vessels in the spinal cord. It results in paralysis of those parts of the body below the blockage, and is frequently mistaken for MS. In addition, SLE can cause thromboses of the small blood vessels in the myelin, or even damage it directly – and damaged myelin is what MS is all about.

Lastly, the whole autoimmune-disease/food-allergy picture leads to a malabsorption of Vitamins B_1, B_3, B_6, B_{12} and folic acid and several important trace elements – all of which are essential to the myelin's health and integrity. As well, the absorption of toxic metals permitted by the food allergies can literally poison the myelin, as it does with so many other body tissues.

You can see what I'm leading up to.

In light of these three family trees, how many people diagnosed as having MS are actually showing some extreme symptoms of autoimmune disease, SLE, food allergies and vitamin-mineral deficiencies? To put it another way, is MS not so much a disease on its own but a combination of all those things, blending them in dreadfully reinforced concert to attack the myelin and severely damage the central nervous system?

In short – are these family trees pointing to a wholly new, tremendously exciting and extraordinarily promising line of research into MS? I believe they are, and that their clues should be followed up without delay.

One way that can be done, of course, is to obtain many more family trees of people with MS. So if you're unlucky enough to have this awful condition in your family, please get busy on your family tree now. You could be a vital partner in this crucial area of medical research and help to bring healing into your family and into thousands of others as well.

Probably MS isn't your problem. Maybe it's cancer, mental illness, diabetes, arthritis, or any one of a thousand other illnesses, mild or serious or in-between.

Whatever it is, please draw up your family tree. Yours could be just the one to provide an essential clue – a clue that could lead to a final breakthrough in the fight against some baffling illness.

Even if its contribution isn't quite so dramatic, it will still do a lot for you and your family. It will identify many factors involved in your present health problem and give you the information you need to overcome them. It will empower you to act against serious illness years before it strikes, and enable you to leave a legacy of health information that will enrich the lives of your children, their children and their children's children after them.

Isn't that worth the cost of a pen, some sheets of paper and a few hours of time?

≈{14}≈

Help for the Hopeless and Hope for the Helpless

SERIOUS ILLNESSES HELPED BY DIET

This chapter is devoted to helping people with auto-immune diseases: their own immune system attacks their tissues and organs, resulting in serious illnesses such as multiple sclerosis (MS), systemic lupus erythematosus (SLE), arthritis, blood vessel disorders and so on.

These illnesses can be killers. They can not only shorten life but they can cause severe pain, paralysis and much anguish for your relatives, your friends and your-self – whether you are a caregiver or a sufferer.

I have come to the conclusions discussed in this chapter after taking the following evidence into account:

- The study of many thousands of detailed health family trees.
- Statistics on food allergies measured on RAST, which is IgE mediated (immediate reaction).
- Statistics on delayed food reactions and chemical sensitivities/intolerances measured by the cytotoxic test, which is not IgE mediated.
- Statistics on antibody reactions measured for gluten and α-gliadin of wheat/gluten-containing grains (delayed sensitivity/intolerance and not IgE mediat-ed) as in celiac disease, etc.
- Statistics on antibody reactions measured for α-casein, α-lactalbumin and β-lactoglobulin of cow's milk (delayed sensitivity/intolerance and not IgE mediated) associated with diabetes, systemic lupus erythematosus (SLE), etc.

240

- Statistics on extensive autoantibody tests (screenings) done to look at antibodies in the tissues and organs, including components of skin, blood vessels, neurological tissues, joints, gut, etc., in key members of many families where autoimmune disease is rampant.
- The study of C3 and C4 complements, which are low in patients with SLE, celiac disease and with sensitivities/intolerances to cow's milk/gluten-containing grains. These complements can also be raised in certain conditions as well.
- Results of measuring immunoglobulins IgA, IgM, IgG, which are types of gamma globulins, and which are high or low in many medical conditions such as celiac disease, SLE, etc.
- Results of tests on immune complexes, which are raised in celiac disease, SLE, etc.
- Results of vitamin assays which show severe deficiencies in vitamins in autoimmune diseases due to malabsorption resulting from cow's milk, gluten-containing grains, legume and bean sensitivities/intolerances. All of these can cause flat gut villi or villous atrophy/destruction. Villi are folds of cells in the gut necessary for the absorption of vitamins and other nutrients.
- Results of mineral assays in serum and on hair analysis, showing severe deficiencies due to the malabsorption as mentioned above.
- Results of tests showing high levels of heavy metals such as lead, copper, mercury and toxic metals such as aluminum in the serum and on hair analysis.
- Results of many other standard tests, including hemoglobin, blood film, fasting blood sugar, thyroid function, liver function and renal function done on thousands of my patients since 1980.

My conclusions from the above evidence are that most autoimmune diseases are primarily dietary and are related to food sensitivities/intolerances, and most can be helped by diet – nutritional intervention – that is, allergy-free diets and correction of their nutrient deficiencies.

Appendix I shows you a special diet that helps stop osteoarthritis or lessen its effects and pain. The same diet, however, will help many other types of autoimmune disease. In general, withdrawing gluten-containing grains, bovine (cow's) dairy products, beef and cane sugar have worked wonders for the overwhelming majority of my patients. While the following information may seem somewhat technical to some readers, I feel that a detailed description of my testing procedures may be helpful to you and to your physician. Therefore, please read on.

OSTEOARTHRITIS This degenerative bone/joint condition is represented diagnostically with positive cartilage antibody testing (also where reticulin antibodies test positive). In treating this condition, the main foods to avoid are gluten-containing grains (such as wheat, rye, oats, corn/maize, buckwheat, millet), cow's milk, beef (dairy products/bovine protein) and cane sugar. In the grains such as wheat, it appears that gluten and α-gliadin are the main fractions/peptides causing damage. In cow's milk it appears to be α-casein, α-lactalbumin and β-lactoglobulin fractions/peptides. However, other components yet to be identified and named may also be causing damage. When avoiding these foods and others showing positive on the cytotoxic test, cartilage and reticulin antibodies become negative. The titres (values) showing on the antibody test typically halve every three months until they show up as negative. Medical supervision is very important, and there should also be supplementation with extra nutrients during this time. Consuming wholegrain bread or cheese or cane sugar thereafter can rapidly result in a flare up of the joints with pain and a return of the cartilage and reticulin antibodies. For some, having cane sugar is like rubbing crushed glass into their joints. Some complain of even worse symptoms with brown/black sugar.

In Australia alone there are over a million osteoarthritis sufferers. People showing positive values for virtually any autoantibody to tissues or organs can benefit from being off cow's milk and gluten-containing grains. When autoimmune disease profiles are done where the person has been totally off cow's milk/cheese for over a year, it is typically very obvious, since very few antibodies to tissues and organs show positive values. This is even more evident when the person has been strictly off gluten-containing grains as well during the same period.

Any person showing any positive antibodies whatsoever should be totally off cow's milk and gluten-containing grains as a start to good health. The presence of antibodies indicates that the body is *fighting itself* in some very specific way as demonstrated by the particular antibodies involved.

The following autoimmune disease conditions do very well with the diet that helps osteoarthritis (see Appendix I) while the associated antibody testing will help identify missed medical conditions, allowing better diagnosis and treatment.

CONNECTIVE TISSUE DISEASES This family of diseases is indicated by positive reticulin antibody testing. Reticulin is a part of the connective tissue in skin, joints, gut, organs, hair follicles (associated with hair loss) whose antibodies are especially raised in celiac disease, multiple sclerosis (MS), motor neuron disease (ALS), Sjogren's Syndrome, systemic lupus (SLE), osteoarthritis, myasthenia gravis, Crohn's disease, ulcerative colitis and many other medical conditions – even in heroin addiction.

GASTRITIS, ULCERS Parietal cells are cells located in the stomach or gastrum. Damage to stomach or gastric cells is called gastritis and is associated with positive parietal antibody test results. The normal value is <1:10, and when a person shows a value of 1:80 upwards, this is usually also associated with raised intrinsic factor antibodies 1:2 (Normal Range <1:2), meaning it is useless. Intrinsic factor is released from a healthy stomach (parietal cells) and is necessary to latch onto B_{12} to form a complex allowing B_{12} to be absorbed in the terminal ileum (the end part of the small bowel before the cecum). The highest levels of intrinsic factor antibodies have been associated with reactions to milk fractions/peptides such as α-casein, α-lactabulin and especially β-lactoglobulin (which also can cause diabetes) rather than gluten or α-gliadin of wheat/gluten-containing grains that also can cause gastritis/parietal cell antibodies to be positive.

The major cause of gastritis and gastric erosions/ulcers is, in my experience, not *Helicobacter pylori* (gastric bacteria), but is due to cow's milk/gluten-containing grain sensitivity/intolerance, and only less often *Helicobacter pylori* infestation, which is often not even present in gastritis patients.

The condition called *pernicious anemia* is due to low levels of vitamin B_{12} where parietal cell antibodies and intrinsic factor antibodies restrict the absorption of the vitamin. It was called *pernicious anemia* in the old days because people actually died from it. These tragic cases were very pale, had anemia, diarrhea, dementia, subacute combined degeneration of the spinal cord, paralysis, premature graying of hair, etc.

It was observed that, if great-grandmother ate raw liver, her health was improved and she did not die. Subsequently, it was discovered that raw liver contained intrinsic factor, and this was the beneficial factor in the liver. Further along the chain of discovery, it was determined that such people had low B_{12}, and when given B_{12} injections, their health dramatically improved. Dr. Barry Marshall identified a gastric bacteria, *Helicobacter pylori*, in the lining of the stomach that can cause erosions, ulcers, gastric cancer and pernicious anemia. My experience, however, is that cow's milk/gluten-containing grains/ celiac disease are typically the real culprits.

PERNICIOUS ANEMIA   This condition is typically indicated by the presence of low B_{12} and intrinsic factor antibodies. I find that it will typically remit when the patient is off of cow's milk (α-casein, α-lactalbumin and especially β-lactoglobulin) and off of gluten-containing grains (gluten, α-gliadin, gliadinomorphin, etc). In addition, *Helicobacter pylori*, if present, needs to be killed off.

Several Nobel Prizes have been awarded for discoveries outlined in this area, and Dr. Marshall most certainly deserves one as well. But I believe that all of these researchers are wrong. The main cause of pernicious anemia is from sensitivity/intolerance to cow's milk (especially β-lactoglobulin) and gluten-containing grains, in addition to (and perhaps as the direct cause of) the *Helicobacter pylori*.

There is an interesting observation for the thousands of patients I have seen since 1980 whose parietal cell antibodies were positive. When rechecked, most have shown these antibodies have become negative as a result of their being off cow's milk and gluten-containing grains – without any treatment of *Helicobacter pylori,* if it was originally present.

It is likely *Helicobacter pylori* bacteria dies off – is starved to death – if it does not have the fractions/peptides of cow's milk/gluten-containing grain it needs to survive! Some gluten-containing grain peptides as small as only seven amino acids, such as gliadinomorphin of wheat and β-casomorphin of β-casein in cow's milk, could possibly end up in the capsule of *Helicobacter pylori*.

The reason that cow's milk/gluten-containing grains apparently cause pernicious anemia erosions, ulcers, gastritis and gastric cancer is possibly due to the carcinogens in cow's milk/gluten-containing grains, which may end up in the capsule of *Helicobacter pylori,* making it carcinogenic also. This theory certainly requires further investigation.

THYROID DISEASE The presence of thyroid antibodies in both thyroglobulin (thyroid hormone) and the microsomal (tissue) of the thyroid gland is called thyroiditis, which simply means an inflammation of the thyroid. A condition called Hashimoto's thyroiditis is associated with *hypothyroidism*, an underactive thyroid. Thyroiditis can also be associated with *hyperthyroidism*, an overactive thyroid. Thyroiditis is known to be associated with celiac disease or gluten-containing grain sensitivity/intolerance. However, it is also very much associated with cow's milk (α-casein, α-lactalbumin and β-lactoglobulin) sensitivity/intolerance, according to my clinical experience. Thyroid antibodies become negative in many cases when cow's milk as well as gluten-containing grains are excluded from the diet.

ADRENAL DISEASE Positive testing for antibodies to the adrenal gland indicates adrenalitis and an increased risk for low cortisol production, Addison's disease/adrenal exhaustion is also often seen with low blood pressure, vitiligo (white dots in skin), proneness to yeast infections, exhaustion, etc. The adrenal antibodies become negative when cow's milk, gluten-containing grains and yeast are removed from the diet. Candida infections (monilia, thrush), if present with the adrenalitis, also need to be controlled.

BREAST CANCER/LUMPS/CYSTS Breast duct antibodies are typically seen in patients with abnormal duct patterns, breast lumps and increased risk for breast cancer. In these individuals, vertical lines in the tips of the fingers (accidental fingerprint patterns of Bierman) are often found, and there is an increased risk for the patient to be B_1 deficient/dependent and to have greater risk for celiac disease or sensitivity/intolerance to gluten-containing grains. There is also a likelihood that the patient will have a Sydney line on one or both palms (i.e. a middle crease that goes right across the palm). This is evidence that the person most likely survived a *threatened miscarriage* when the nerve networks in the hands, early in fetal development, were affected. This could be due to low vitamin B_1 or vitamin B_6, causing the palmar creases above these nerve networks to be affected. It is known from one survey that women with breast cancer showed a greater incidence of accidental fingerprint patterns of Bierman, [i.e., 250/1000 (25%) for breast cancer as compared to only 6/1000 (.6%) from the normal population]. People developing breast cancer as adults are often born with abnormal duct patterns. Where the breast cancer is familial, the patient's skin is also typically different: plated fibroblasts behave like fetal fibroblasts – not adult fibroblasts. Such abnormalities of fingerprint patterns, palmar creases, duct patterns and even skin matrix suggest *transplacental induction* of breast cancer – that is, it formed as a type of congenital abnormality most likely at a time of threatened miscarriage due to disturbances in levels of vitamins, minerals, and hormones such as DHEA (dehydroepiandrosterone).

THREATENED MISCARRIAGE AND CANCER It is known that as fetal DHEA falls, the mother's placental release of estrogens to maintain the fetus (baby) diminishes, and miscarriage can result.

In the first edition of this book and in lectures I have given subsequently, I predicted that certain cancer cells, as in breast cancer, would be shown to have receptors not only for hormones such as estrogens and androgens, but also for food peptides or fractions called *lectins*. I theorized that these lectins also could have estrogenlike activity and that breast cancer cells could possibly also have receptors for herbicides or pesticides with estrogenlike activity.

Today, it is known that breast cancer can have receptors for hormones and the food fractions called lectins. It
is also known that melanoma, another condition that is
transplacentally induced (i.e., a congenital abnormality
that people are born with), can have receptors for certain
glycoproteins (lectins) of peanuts. And it is now known
that certain pesticides can concentrate in specific cancer
tissues as in the case of pancreatic cancer. The question
thus arises: **Are most cancers a result of the patient
having survived a threatened miscarriage and having
been born with precancerous tissue?**

According to this theory, the moles people are born
with may have the potential to become malignant
melanoma later in life, polyps to become stomach or
bowel cancer; abnormal breast-duct patterns, skin layer-
ing, palmar creases to manifest as breast cancer; abnormal bone marrow to become leukemia later on, and so
on. Notably, children born with Down's Syndrome have
what is genetically called *trisomy 21* (three 21 chromosomes instead of two) and are more at risk to be born
with leukemia. Other children can also have trisomy 21,
but only in cells in the bone marrow or other aneuplodies
(chromosomal abnormalities), making them very much
at risk for leukemia later.

Even patients with bowel cancer have abnormal bow-
els compared with a person without bowel cancer. The
apparently normal bowel tissues, isolated from the bowel
cancer in a cancer patient, stain differently (different
isoenzymes) compared with tissue from a control bowel
in an individual without cancer. Thus, the apparently
normal tissue is not normal, and the bowel is actually different – a type of congenital abnormality where polyps
are found in the stomach or bowel and some intestinal
cells appear in the stomach, causing a risk for stomach
cancer later on.

In my theory of transplacental induction of stomach
cancer (1974) see references at the end of the book),
I had thought the children with risk for gastric cancer

were born with precancerous cells in the stomach and some intestinal cells that should not be there from faulty differentiation at time of threatened miscarriage. However, it is now known that Helicobacter can cause damage in the stomach of animals and gastritis, erosions and then ulcers and then later malignant changes and *intestinalization of the stomach* where intestinal cells appear in the stomach.

This suggests an additional clue to gastric cancer development *in utero*. The following questions spring to mind: Can *Helicobacter pylori* pass across the placenta and end up in the fetal parietal (stomach) cells and act as a carcinogen, causing the intestinalization of the stomach and premalignant changes? Has *Helicobacter pylori* been found in the fetal stomach of children who have been miscarried? Do small fractions of cow's milk such as β-casomorphin (only seven amino acids long) and small fractions of wheat/gluten-containing grains such as gliadinomorphin (also only seven amino acids long) act as carcinogens, passing across the placenta and affecting the vulnerable developing fetal stomach at critical periods in fetal differentiation (formation)? If these peptides/fractions (potential carcinogens) from milk/grains can also end up in the capsule of *Helicobacter pylori*, then is this why it is carcinogenic?

If a fetus has a stomach with polyps and intestinal cells in it that should not be there normally, and no evidence of *Helicobacter pylori*, or if Helicobacter is too large to pass across the placental barrier, then it is just the small milk and gluten-containing grain fractions that are causing the intestinalization of the stomach (precancer, etc.).

All the above certainly supports the idea that the person most at risk for bowel cancer is born with a very different bowel than that of a healthy individual, a bowel with polyps in the stomach, perhaps intestinal cells in the stomach and polyps in the bowel, and with completely different enzymes in the gut, called *isoenzymes*.

MS – TRANSPLACENTALLY INDUCED? From my clinical research, another transplacentally induced condition is MS, likely because over 50% of my MS patients have a Sydney line on their left hand, suggesting they have survived a threatened miscarriage. This is a strong indication that they were born with abnormal plaques in their brain or spinal cord, which later developed into the disease. It is known that patients who will later develop MS can have these plaques (silent MS) for years before manifesting the disease. Thus, are MS plaques formed in the fetus at a time of threatened miscarriage while the fetus is low in B_1, B_6, biotin, DHEA estrogens, etc. (most likely essential for normal fetal neurological tissue development), and at critical periods of differentiation/formation of these neurological tissues?

OTHER TRANSPLACENTAL INDUCTIONS Similarly, can uterine cancer be transplacentally induced? One patient with uterine cancer confirmed that her mother had two miscarriages before her and one miscarriage after her and nearly lost her due to a threatened miscarriage. When uterine cancer was detected in her womb, there was also a polyp and a fibroid, showing evidence that she possibly was born with precancerous tissue and the other two conditions as well.

Men with accidental fingerprint patterns of Bierman are also much more at risk to develop prostate cancer – again supporting transplacental induction of cancer.

If low fetal DHEAS can cause miscarriage or threatened miscarriage, it is little wonder that low DHEAS in later life would increase the risk for cancer, MS, CNS degeneration and other problems. And in fact it has now been shown that low DHEA increases the risk for many types of cancer and that DHEA (acting like cortisone, yet without its side effects) can help MS patients.

It is also my observation in patients with MS, motor neuron disease, Huntington's chorea, cerebellar atrophy and cancer that they are very likely to be low in DHEAS.

The good news is that a positive test for breast duct antibodies can be reversed by removing cow's milk, gluten-
containing grains, and all other foods and chemicals to
which the person is sensitive from their diet, thereby
stopping chronic inflammation and the release of PGE2
series, tumor necrosis factor a (TNFa) and other cytokines
that can flare up cancer.

PROSTATITIS, PROSTATE CANCER Prostrate antibody development can be triggered, according to my clinical experience, by cow's milk and gluten-containing grains.
Removing these elements from their diet has been
tremendously helpful to my patients with prostatitis,
prostatic hypertrophy and prostate cancer.

From the information presented above, men with a
history of prostate cancer in their family and with heavy
vertical lines in the tips of their fingers should have their
PSA checked and monitored regularly. If raised, other
tests should be performed to followup on the possibility
of cancer of the prostate, hypertrophy, etc.

When breast and prostate cancer is added to the family health tree, it becomes obvious that mothers with
breast cancer are more likely to have sons with prostate
cancer. And men who have prostate cancer are more
likely to have daughters with breast cancer. Both have
an increased incidence for the presence of accidental
fingerprint patterns of Bierman (vertical lines in the tips
of fingers). Why? Could it be due to celiac disease,
which in my experience is associated with low B_1, somehow causing these problems? I have recorded palmar
creases and nutrient deficiencies in over five thousand
patients now.

Future research workers in this area will be looking
for similar carcinogens in gluten-containing grains and
in cow's milk that can pass across the placenta and act
like hormones causing abnormal differentiation and
laying down receptors for these carcinogens in various
precancerous tissues.

THE LEAKY PLACENTA SYNDROME I would like to introduce to you a concept that I believe is new – *the leaky placenta syndrome*. The *leaky gut syndrome* is now well accepted. This occurs where undigested food peptides/lectins/carcinogens not normally passing across the villi/gut wall do pass across. The increased permeability of the gut wall is due to the loss of intestinal villi – in celiac disease as well as with cow's milk and legume and bean sensitivity/intolerance and with *Candida Albicans* infestation.

It is known that umbilical cord blood can show positive to cow's milk and gluten-containing grains on the cytotoxic test. This means the child can be sensitized to these foods **across the placenta**. Is there a group of pregnant women who because of leaky placenta syndrome pass far more food fractions/peptides/lectins/exorphins (opioidlike peptides such as gliadinomorphin of α-gliadin of wheat, etc., and β-casomorphin of β-casein of cow's milk, etc.) and pesticides, herbicides, bacteria, candida, viruses and other agents to the developing fetus? If this is the case, far more mutagens (causing mutations in genes), teratogens (causing congenital abnormalities), carcinogens (causing cancer later), and food peptides and chemicals causing food and chemical sensitivity/intolerance in the child would result. This also would apply to carcinogenic changes in the fetal stomach, potentially manifesting later in life as stomach cancer – especially with a further *Helicobacter pylori* infestation. Is it possible that cervical (womb) human papillomavirus (wart virus) can pass across the placenta in some women and cause precancerous changes to the fetus *in utero*?

Appendix (L) shows you a family with a mother who went gray by the age of thirty (most likely a celiac) with twelve daughters who developed cancer. The middle ten all had cancer of the uterus (womb) – did a wart papillomavirus initiate precancerous changes – cause some mutations/chromosomal changes in certain vulnerable tissues at critical periods of uterine tissue differentiation (formation)?

Where do the mutagens, teratogens, carcinogens, food peptides/lectins, and others. come from? The most likely answer to that is that the mother has leaky gut syndrome and has these in her own blood during pregnancy. Correction of celiac disease and other causes of leaky gut syndrome should take place before becoming pregnant and especially during pregnancy, and this may stop leaky placenta syndrome with its devastating effects on the unborn child.

DIABETES Islet-cell antibody formation of autoimmune diabetes may be triggered by cow's milk and gluten-containing grains.

It is well known that diabetes is one of over a hundred illnesses associated with celiac disease (gluten, α-gliadin sensitivity/intolerance, etc.). Both β-lactoglobulin and especially β-casein sensitivity/intolerance can be associated with autoimmune diabetes, especially juvenile diabetes.

NEPHRITIS This inflammation of the kidney basement membrane is indicated clinically by positive testing for glomerular antibodies. Nephrons are the filtering parts of the kidneys. If these are damaged, the kidneys can pass high amounts of protein in the urine. This is called proteinuria. In acute glomerulonephritis (kidney infection/ inflammation), the blood passed in the urine is called *hematuria* and the result can be kidney failure with the need for a kidney transplant.

Nephritis of the kidney as an autoimmune disease is seen in many other conditions – especially diabetes, SLE and celiac disease. Again it is wise to totally avoid cow's milk, cheese, dairy products and the grains containing both gluten and especially α-gliadin – more toxic than gluten (and a part of gluten).

There is a type of glomerulonephritis specifically due to α-gliadin of wheat/ gluten-containing grains that can be helped by being on a gluten- (α-gliadin-) free diet. Many people with this condition can still have a normal bowel biopsy. Whether or not a biopsy of the small bowel is done (confirming villous atrophy/destruction), all people with classical celiac disease or α-gliadin sensitivity/intolerance need to be off gluten (and the α-gliadin in it) for the rest of their lives. This will decrease their risk of developing malignancies, including: leukemia, bowel cancer, breast cancer, prostate cancer, ovarian cancer, uterine (womb) cancer, gastric cancer, pancreatic cancer, etc., and will decrease their risk of developing osteoarthritis, diabetes, dementia/Alzheimer's disease, etc.

CHRONIC FATIGUE: MYOSITIS, MYALGIA, MYOSTHENIA GRAVIS AND THYMOMA Antireceptor antibodies are seen with skeletal muscle antibodies in the inflammation of voluntary muscle tissue called *myositis* or *myalgia*. These antibodies are also seen with myasthenia gravis – a condition where the eyelids often droop (ptosis) and where the muscles tire very rapidly and the person can become too weak to do such a task as hang clothes out on a clothesline to dry.

This condition can also be associated with a thymoma – a tumor of the thymus gland. It can also be seen in celiac disease and with cow's milk sensitivity/intolerance. In my patients with these conditions, I have typically witnessed the antibodies reverse to negative on a diet free of cow's milk and gluten-containing grains.

A neurological diagnosis is generally helpful. Eaton-Lambert Syndrome, due to cancer of the lung, is a disease that can mimic myasthenia gravis and needs to be considered. Myasthenia gravis can also be associated with a positive test for reticulin antibodies as described previously. The presence of these antibodies is diagnostic for cow's milk/gluten-containing-grain sensitivity/intolerance, and will reverse to negative when the patient removes these particular foods from their diet.

INFLAMMATION OF THE OVARIES, OVARIAN CANCER Antiovary antibodies indicate an inflammation of the ovary called o-ophoritis. This condition can cause the ovary to become atrophied and nonfunctional with time and can result in premature menopause or diminished estrogen production. In my experience with familial cancer patients, antiovary antibodies indicate an increased risk for ovarian cancer.

Ovarian atrophy in alcoholics is not only due to their increased risk for low B_1 (thiamin) but also because their higher intake of malt, barley and yeast extracts makes them more likely to manufacture reticulin antibodies and ovary antibodies to their own detriment.

Infertility is very common in celiacs, and celiac mothers are highly at risk to miscarry and are more at risk to have Down's Syndrome children, it would appear from my research. I regard untreated celiac disease with its hundred or so associated illnesses, manifesting prior to conception, as the major cause of Down's Syndrome. This is particularly so if the woman is low in B_1, B_3, B_6, Vitamin C, biotin, and other nutrients. Spina bifida, cleft palate and harelip can also be seen in the children of celiac mothers, particularly when these women are low in iron and folic acid as a result of malabsorbing these nutrients. Future research may confirm my suspicion that low biotin levels prior to conception may be a cause for Klinefelter's Syndrome (XXY) when a male has an extra X chromosome and is born with undeveloped testes, a condition called hypogonadism. This condition has been seen in animals made low in biotin during pregnancy. (See reference 11 at the end of the book)

Biotin, B_3, B_6, Vitamin C, magnesium, zinc, manganese and selenium are important to help convert g-linolenic acid to the essential PGE1 hormone series (first messenger), necessary for normal meiosis or cell division of the ova. Normal cell division prevents chromosomal abnormalities (aneuplodies) such as Trisomy 21 (Down's Syndrome) and XO (Turner's Syndrome) and XXY (Klinefelter's Syndrome). Vitamins B_1, B_3, C, calcium and magnesium are important for forming cAMP (second messenger) and are also important for meiosis and other cell-division mechanisms.

Untreated celiac disease with the above nutrient deficiencies, risk for hypothyroidism and risk for low DHEA hormone prior to conception is, in my opinion, a *disaster waiting to happen*. Untreated celiac disease in pregnancy is also a major cause of nausea and vomiting due to low levels of vitamins B_1, B_6, biotin, etc. Combined with low DHEA, these can result in miscarrriage, since it is known that as fetal DHEAS falls, the placental estrogens also fall – as is typically seen with an imminent miscarriage. (See Appendix L.)

Another problem in pregnancy caused or aggravated by celiac disease is gestational diabetes, which may be due to low vitamin B_6, biotin, etc. Vitamin B_6 (pyridoxal) has been successfully used to treat gestational diabetes. Biotin can act like insulin. In the past, many women took Debendox for nausea/vomiting of pregnancy since it contained B_6. If nausea and vomiting of pregnancy is severe and life threatening, intramuscular injection of vitamin B_1 (thiamin) can help. It is known that toxemia of pregnancy can be helped by vitamins B_1, B_6, Vitamin C, magnesium, zinc, etc., and it is known that celiac disease can cause all these deficiencies, as well as cause other nutrients to be low.

CONGENITAL ABNORMALITIES It is unfortunate that women needing epileptic drugs before and during pregnancy are more likely to have children with congenital abnormalities. One major reason for this is that the women can be low in folic acid. As celiac disease is a major cause of low folic acid, iron, etc., it should not be a surprise that it is a major cause, if untreated, of congenital abnormalities in children and can be associated with spina bifida, cleft palate, harelip and anencephaly (child born with no skull or with brain exposed). Animals made low in B-group vitamins can be born with severe congenital abnormalities of limbs, paws, etc. The drug Thalidomide can also cause severe deformities of limbs, hands, feet, etc. Thalidomide can cause a sensory neuropathy (nerve damage). The treatment for exposure to this drug – B-group vitamins!

Children of diabetic mothers can be born with thalidomidelike deformities even though the mothers were not on thalidomide. Why? Could it be that diabetics, especially those with celiac disease, tend to be similarly low in B-group vitamins, including B_1, B_6, biotin, folic acid, and iron, and are also at risk to have low DHEAS? It is known that low DHEAS increases the risk for diabetes, and celiacs are also more at risk for low DHEAS.

I find it fascinating that during my research into the causes of congenital defects in Down's Syndrome, I have seen the beneficial effects of B-group vitamin supplementation. Mothers who have conceived a Down's Syndrome child, but taken B-group vitamins during their pregnancies, have borne children who do so much better than usual and look far less like a Down's Syndrome child than those who have not taken these nutrients. Such a Down's Syndrome child has relatively low-grade abnormalities and can have normal little fingers with two creases rather than one, and not have the usual hole in the heart. Other Down's Syndrome children usually have severe congenital abnormalities of the heart and can have holes in the heart, needing to be surgically closed, and their hands can show Sydney lines or simian palmar creases with one crease replacing the usual two that go right across the palm.

Other children can have all of the above phenotypes, or appearances, of Down's Syndrome, but not the Karyotype – the extra chromosome 21, called Trisomy 21, indicating the person is a Down's Syndrome child. Why? It is not necessarily the extra chromosome 21 that causes the congenital abnormalities – it is something else – and I believe this is severe B-group vitamin deficiencies and celiac disease. In my studies of mothers with children showing short little fingers with one crease only in the little fingers and a hole in the heart, the one nutrient deficiency that is most common is vitamin B_1. Of interest, when children are born with holes in the heart (defective walls) and there is correction of their B-group vitamin deficiencies (particularly B_1 and B_6) this has often resulted in the holes closing, much to the surprise of the pediatrician looking after the children.

BACK TO THE FAMILY TREE   When you draw up your family health tree, record such things as abnormal palmar creases, diabetes, celiac disease, miscarriages, nausea/ vomiting of pregnancy, gestational diabetes (sugar in the urine), toxemia of pregnancy (with high blood pressure, fitting and protein in the urine), crib deaths (low B_6 more likely than low B_1, biotin, Vitamin C, selenium, etc.) and congenital abnormalities such as short little fingers, holes in the heart, heart defects, harelip, cleft palate, anencephaly, spina bifida, thalidomidelike deformities and the chromosomal abnormalities I have mentioned above.

Recording blood group (such as A, B, O, AB) and whether Rh is positive or negative is worth doing. There are excellent books suggesting food groups that are healthier for these specific blood types.

However, when autoimmune disease is present, it is wise to have tests done to look for gluten, α-gliadin sensitivity/intolerance, celiac disease, cow's milk sensitivity/intolerance and other sensitivities/intolerances that can show on the cytotoxic test and on RAST, both IgE (immediate) and IgG (delayed) reactions.

In some families there are other blood groups that should also be recorded. These include HLA blood type – HLA-B27 is seen with ankylosing spondylitis; HLA-B8 with celiac disease and SLE; HLA DRW3 where the person has seventy times the usual risk for celiac disease and also an increased risk for dermatitis herpetiformis (due to gluten and α-gliadin sensitivity/intolerance), insulin dependent diabetes mellitus (*juvenile diabetes*), thyroiditis, adrenalitis, etc.

People with HLA DRW3 are also more at risk for full-blown AIDS, to have suffered from toxic rapeseed syndrome in Spain, EMS (eosinophilic myalgic syndrome) in the USA from contaminated/genetically engineered L-tryptophan poisoning (bad batch), and have risk for SLE and coxsacchie B virus infections (which can also cause diabetes).

Why?

It appears there is a genetic susceptibility for sensitivity/intolerance to glycoproteins and toxic peptides of gluten-containing grains, yeast, viral and bacterial capsules and pollens (called pollinosis).

If HLA DRW3 tests positive, whatever the illness associated, be it celiac disease, SLE, AIDS (see reference 26) or juvenile diabetes, it would appear very wise to exclude gluten-containing grains and yeast from the diet and check for *Candida albicans* (monilia, thrush) and other opportunist pathogens (containing toxic glycoproteins) so these "bugs" can be treated to help reduce the autoimmune disease present.

To summarize:

Nutritional Intervention to help autoimmune diseases: A cow's milk/gluten-free diet

The following antibodies to various tissues/organs can be dramatically reduced by removing cow's milk (dairy products), gluten-containing grains, cane sugar and, ideally, yeast from the patient's diet:

- Cartilage antibodies (seen in osteoarthritis)
- Reticulin antibodies (seen in celiac disease, Sjogrens Syndrome, Crohn's disease, myasthenia gravis, multiple sclerosis (MS), motor neurone disease (ALS), ulcerative colitis, and many other medical conditions and in heroin addiction)
- Parietal cell antibodies (seen in gastritis and/or *Helicobacter pylori* infestation)
- Intrinsic factor antibodies (seen in pernicious anemia and risk for low B_{12})
- Thyroid antibodies (seen in thyroiditis)
- Adrenal antibodies (seen in adrenalitis)

- Breast duct antibodies (seen with breast lumps, breast cancer risk, etc.)
- Prostate antibodies (seen with prostatitis, prostate hypertrophy and risk for prostate cancer)
- Islet cell antibodies (juvenile diabetes, etc.)
- Glomerular antibodies (seen in glomerulonephritis as in celiac disease, diabetes, SLE, etc.)
- Antireceptor antibodies (seen in myasthenia gravis)
- Ovary antibodies (seen with o-ophoritis/inflammation of ovary and with risk for ovarian cancer)

OTHER AUTOIMMUNE DISEASES NEEDING SPECIAL DIETS TO REVERSE

There are two special diets I have devised over the years that have helped thousands of patients with various autoimmune diseases. They are:

1. SLE-reversing diet, which includes being off cow's milk, beef, eggs, gluten-containing grains, legumes, beans, cane sugar and yeast. (See Appendix J.)

2. Synovitis-reversing diet, which involves being off the above foods and also citrus, solanaceae and salicylate-rich foods as well. (See Appendix K.)

SLE-REVERSING DIET

The antibodies to various tissues and organs that can be reversed by this diet are as follows:

1. ANF (antinuclear factor)
2. ds DNA (double-stranded DNA) ⎬ seen in systemic lupus erythematosus (SLE).
3. lymphocyte antibodies
4. Smooth-muscle antibodies, indicating acute or chronic active hepatitis and vasculitis (also need to kill off *Chlamydia pneumonia*, an opportunist pathogen, if present).
5. Bile duct antibodies of cholangitis (inflammation of lining of bile ducts in the liver).
6. Colon antibodies of colitis such as ulcerative colitis.

7. Pancreatic duct antibodies with risk for diabetes.
8. Antinerve antibodies } of multiple sclerosis (MS).
9. Antimyelin antibodies } and other neurological conditions.
10. Anti-GM1 ganglioside antibodies } of motor neuron
    disease (ALS).
11. Anterior horn cell antibodies   } and other neurological
    conditions.
12. Antimeninges antibodies of meningioma, etc.
    Combinations of 8 to 12 (antibodies to neurological tis-
    sues) can occur with multiple sclerosis and motor neurone
    disease (ALS). With these autoimmune neuritis conditions,
    the following opportunist pathogens need to be identified
    and killed off, if present:

    • *Candida albicans* (thrush, monilia).

    • *Chlamydia pneumonia,* also seen commonly with smooth-
      muscle antibodies of vasculitis (arteriosclerosis), and
      with chronic cough, pneumonia, pleurisy, asthma,
      hypertension, pericarditis, cardiomyopathy and in
      multiple sclerosis (MS) and motor neuron disease (ALS).

    • *Campylobacter jejuni* (especially in motor neurone
      disease/ALS, showing GM1 ganglioside antibodies posi-
      tive). Also, in MS and ALS, they must not remain low in
      B_1, B_3, B_6, B_{12}, folic acid, etc., to maintain myelin, etc.
      (See Appendix G.)

13. Melanocyte antibodies indicating risk for vitiligo
    (depigmented areas of skin).
14. Skeletal muscle antibodies
15. Tropomyosin muscle-fiber antibodies   seen with
                                                  myositis, myalgia,
16. Actin muscle-fiber antibodies   fibromyalgia,
                                                  myopathies.
17. Actinomyosin muscle-fiber antibodies

Note*: Skeletal muscle, antireceptor, reticulin antibodies
positive suggest myasthenia gravis.*

SYNOVITIS-REVERSING DIET

There are many serious illnesses that can be helped by this diet.

The antibodies that can be reversed by this diet are as follows

1. ANCA antibodies of   – polyarteritis nodosa
   – Wegeners granulomatosis
   – inflammatory arthritis
   – blood vessel disorders (vasculitis)

2. Rheumatoid factor of rheumatoid arthritis.

3. Synovial membrane antibodies of synovitis

4. Elastin antibodies of elastinitis

5. Collagen antibodies of collagenitis

6. Fibrin antibodies of fibrinitis

    seen with rheumatoid arthritis, synovitis, scleroderma, Sjogren's Syndrome, ankylozing spondylitis vasculitis, etc.,

7. Endothelium antibodies of vasculitis (inflammation of lining of vessels).

8. Mitochondrial antibodies of primary biliary cirrhosis

9. Collagen antibodies and antinerve antibodies of neurofibromatosis

10. Bladder epithelium antibodies of allergic trigonitis and cystitis.

11. Cardiolipin antibodies as in SLE.

12. Conjunctival antibodies in conjuntivitis.

Note: *Cancer patients should be on a similar diet, but also need to be off all meats, poultry and their fats, and have filtered water and organic foods, where possible, to help exclude pesticides, herbicides, etc.*

APPENDIX A

Illnesses, categorized for family trees

Blood disorders
Cancers
Cardiovascular (heart & blood vessels)
Endocrine (glandular)
Eye disorders
Gastrointestinal
Gynecological
Immunological
Infections
Neurological/psychiatric
Renal (kidney)
Respiratory
Skeleto-muscular
Skin disorders

BLOOD DISORDERS

anemia
aplastic anemia
blood group
cholesterol – low, raised
circulation poor
clotting/coagulation disorder
cortisol – low (Addison's disease), raised (Cushing's Syndrome)
familial – hyperbilirubinemia (raised bile), hypercalcaemia (raised calcium), hyperlipoproteinemia (raised lipids: fats)
folic acid deficiency
hemophilia
hyperinsulinemia (raised insulin)

hypoglycemia (low blood sugar)
iron deficiency anemia
leucocytosis (increased white cells)
leukemia – acute, granulocytic, lymphoblastic, lymphatic, lymphocytic, myeloblastic, myelogenous, nonlymphoblastic
macrocytic anemia (low vitamins B_1, B_{12}, folate, etc.)
macrocytosis (enlarged red cells)
Mediterranean anemia
myeloma (multiple)
newborn, hemolytic disease of
nevus (birth mark)
pernicious anemia

263

phenylketonuria (PKU: mental
retardation)
platelet – coagulation defects,
deficiency
polycythemia (opposite of
anemia)
pyridoxine (B_6) deficiency
causing convulsions or
sideroblastic anemia
RH blood group
riboflavin deficiency (B_2)
sickle cell anemia
thalassemias (Mediterranean
anemia)
uremia (raised urea)
vitamin B_{12} deficiency
vitamin K deficiency
Von Willebrand's disease
(bleeding disorder)

CANCERS

basal cell carcinoma (skin
cancers on face)
bone tumor
bowel cancer
brain cancer
brain tumor
breast cancer
bronchial cancer (lung)
cervical cancer (womb)
duodenal cancer
eye cancer
islet-cell tumors (pancreas)
laryngeal cancer (larynx)
lip carcinoma
liver cancer
lung cancer
lymphomas
melanoma (malignant mole)
metastases (secondary cancer
from a primary)

multiple myeloma (cancer of
bone)
neck cancer
nose tumors
osteosarcoma (cancer of bone)
ovarian carcinoma
pancreas carcinoma
pharyngeal carcinoma
prostatic cancer
rectum carcinoma
seminomas (cancer of testes)
sigmoid cancer (lower bowel)
tongue carcinoma
tonsil carcinoma
vaginal carcinoma
vocal cord carcinoma

CARDIOVASCULAR (HEART AND BLOOD VESSELS)

aorta coarctation (narrowing)
aortic – aneurysm, incompe-
tence (weak valves, stenosis
(narrowing of valves)
arrhythmias (irregular heart beats)
arteriosclerosis (hardening of
arteries)
arterio venous fistula (join
between arteries and veins)
atrial – fibrillation (very rapid
heart beat), septal defect
(congenital heart defect)
beri beri (low B_1)
berry aneurysm
cardiac failure
cardiomyopathy (disease of
heart muscle)
carotid artery – aneurysm
(dilation), stenosis (blockage)
coronary artery thrombosis
embolism pulmonary (blood
clot in lung)

essential hypertension (high
blood pressure)
heart valve failure
infarction (blockage) – heart,
brain or lungs
ischemia (narrowing of vessels)
heart or brain
Marfan's Syndrome
murmurs
myocarditis (inflammation of
heart covering)
pericarditis (inflammation of
heart covering)
phlebitis (inflammation of
veins)
piles (hemorrhoids)
Raynaud's disease (purple hands
when cold)
rheumatic fever
SLE (systemic lupus
erythematosus)
stroke (CVA, cerebral hemorrhage or thrombosis)
subarachnoid hemorrhage
(bleeding into brain)
thrombosis (clot) artery, vein
varicose veins of legs,
esophagus, testes
xanthomatosis (fatty plaques
around eyes).

ENDOCRINE/GLANDULAR

Addison's disease (adrenal gland
failure)
adenitis (swollen glands)
adrenal gland disorders
Cushing's Syndrome (raised
cortisol)
diabetes insipidus
diabetes mellitus
gigantism (acromegaly)

goiter
Grave's disease (overactive
thyroid)
juvenile diabetes
ovarian dermoid cyst (tumors)
parathyroid – overactive,
underactive
pituitary gland – adenoma
(tumor), overactive,
underactive
prostate disease
testes – absent, infertility,
Klinefelter's Syndrome
thyroid cancer

EYE DISORDERS

astigmatism
color-blind
conjunctivitis
cornea (ulcers, kerato conus)
dislocated lens (Marfan's
Syndrome)
iritis (inflammation of iris)
optic atrophy
proptosis (protruding eyes)
retina pigmentary degeneration
retinitis (inflammation of retina)
retrobulbar neuritis (damaged
nerve behind eye)
strabismus (squint)
sty (hordeolum)
vision – double, impaired
vitamin A deficiency

GASTROINTESTINAL

achlorhydria (lack of gastric
juices)
anal fissure
appendicitis
biliary – cirrhosis, colic (gall
bladder pain)

bowel tumor
calculus (stone) – gall bladder,
    kidney, salivary gland duct
cholecystitis (gall bladder
    inflammation)
cirrhosis of liver
celiac disease
colon disorder
colostomy (for obstruction,
    bowel cancer)
cystic fibrosis
diverticulitis
duodenal ulcer
familial polyposis of bowel
    (bowel polyp)
gall bladder disease
gallstones
gastritis
gastoenteritis
gluten sensitivity – enteropathy,
    celiac disease
hemorrhoids
hepatomas (liver tumor)
hiatus hernia
ileitis regional (Crohn's disease)
intestinal obstruction
intussusception (telescoping of
    bowel)
malabsorption syndrome
malnutrition
megacolon (enlarged colon)
mesenteric adenitis (enlarged
    glands in abdomen)
milk intolerance (lactase
    enzyme deficiency)
mucous colitis
overweight (obesity)
pancreatitis
parotid gland cyst
parotitis (mumps)
pelvic abscess
peptic ulcer (gastric, duodenal)

peritonitis
Peutz-Jegher's Syndrome (brown
    spots on lips and bowel
    polyps)
polyps, bowel
proctitis (inflammation in anal
    area)
pyloric stenosis
pyorrhea alveolaris
rectal fissure
spastic colon
spleen atrophy
splenomegaly (enlarged spleen)
stomach – polyps, ulcer
ulcerative colitis
wheat gluten intolerance/celiac
    disease

GYNECOLOGICAL

ante partum hemorrhage
    (prebirth bleeding)
big babies (mother at risk for
    diabetes later)
breast cancer
breast cysts
breast lumps
breech delivery
candidiasis (thrush/monilia)
cysts – breast, ovaries
eclampsia (fits while pregnant)
ectopic pregnancy
endometriosis (chocolate cysts)
fibrocystic disease of breast
    (lumps)
mastitis (inflammation of breast)
menorrhagia (heavy periods)
menstruation – absence,
    premenstrual tension
miscarriage
ovarian – abscess, cysts
placenta previa (placenta
    blocking birth)

polycystic disease of ovary
polyps – endometrial (womb or
    uterus)
postpartum hemorrhage
    (postbirth bleeding)
pregnancy – iron deficiency
    anemia (craving ice)
    – irregular vaginal bleeding
       (threatened miscarriage)
    – nausea and vomiting
    – perverted appetite
    – perverted taste
puerperal depression ("baby blues")
salpingitis (infected Fallopian
    tubes)
threatened abortion (TMC)
toxemia of pregnancy (high
    blood pressure)
trichomonas vaginitis
uterine – fibroids, polyps
vaginal abnormalities
vaginal discharges
vaginitis

IMMUNOLOGICAL

allergy
angioneurotic edema (face and
    hands puff up)
autoimmune disease
cervical adenopathy (swollen
    glands in neck)
coryza (hay fever)
food allergy/intolerance
Hodgkin's disease (cancer of
    lymph nodes)
immunodeficiency diseases (born
    with very high infection risks)

INFECTIONS

AIDS
amoebic dysentery
bacillary dysentery

Born Holm's disease (chest pain
    after virus)
chicken pox
cholera
diphtheria
ear (middle) infections
encephalitis
flu (influenza)
fungal infections
giardiasis (parasite causing diar-
    rhea)
gonorrhea
Hansen's disease (leprosy)
hepatitis viral – A infectious, B
    serum
herpes – simplex, zoster
hydatid cysts
mononucleosis (glandular fever)
malaria
measles
meningitis
monilia (thrush, candida
    albicans)
mumps
neurosyphilis
parasites
paronychia (fungal infections of
    the nail)
plantar wart
poliomyelitis
scarlet fever
septicemia (blood poisoning)
sexually transmitted diseases –
    gonorrhea, syphilis
shingles (herpes zoster)
staphylococcal infections
streptococcal infections
typhoid fever
venereal disease
viral hepatitis
whooping cough (pertussis)

Neurological/psychiatric

acoustic neuroma (tumor on
   auditory nerve)
addiction
alcoholism
Alzheimer's disease
amyotrophic lateral sclerosis
   (ALS)
anorexia nervosa (slimmers'
   disease)
anxiety state
autism
barbiturate addiction
behavior disorders
Bell's palsy (facial nerve paralysis)
blackouts
brain abscess
burning-feet syndrome
carpal tunnel syndrome (pains
   in wrist)
cataplexy (tendency to collapse)
cerebellum disorders (affecting
   balance)
cerebral palsy (spasticity)
cigarette smoking addiction
conduction deafness
Creutzfeldt-Jacob disease
demyelinating disease (such as MS)
epilepsy
epiloia (mental retardation with
   fits)
familial mental retardation
familial periodic paralysis
familial tremor
glioma (brain tumor)
grand mal epilepsy
Huntington's chorea
intermittent acute porphyria
leucotomy (brain surgery for
   depression)
manic-depressive psychosis

mastoiditis
Meniere's disease
mental retardation
mongolism (Down's Syndrome)
motor neuron disease (ALS/amy-
   otrophic lupus sclerosis)
multiple sclerosis
myasthenia gravis (lassitude,
   muscle weakness)
myoclonic epilepsy
nerve deafness
neurodermatitis
neurofibromatosis (tumors on
   nerves)
neuropathy peripheral (wrist,
   foot drop)
neurosis (chronic anxiety state)
niacin deficiency (pellagra)
paraplegia (congenital)
Parkinson's disease
petit mal epilepsy
polyneuropathy (damage to
   nerves – many causes)
porphyria
presenile dementia
psychomotor epilepsy (temporal
   lobe epilepsy)
quadriplegia (congenital)
sciatica
seizures
senile dementia
spinal cord – degeneration, tumors
status epilepticus
Sturge-Weber disease (port wine
   stain on face, damage to brain)
subacute combined degeneration
   of spinal cord (due to low
   Vitamin B_{12}/pernicious anemia)
subdural hematoma (bleeding
   into brain cavity)
syringomyelia (slow paralysis)

thiamine deficiency (beri beri)
thiamine – Wernicke's disease
  (severe Vitamin B$_1$ deficiency)
tic douloureux
tremor familial
von Recklinghausen's disease
zoster (herpes)

RENAL (KIDNEY)

Bright's disease (kidney failure)
cystinosis
cystinuria
cystitis recurrent (bladder
  infection)
glomerulonephritis
glucosuria (glucose in urine)
homocystinuria
irritable bladder
kidney – carcinoma, ectopic,
  failure, stones
nephrogenic diabetes insipidus
pyelitis, pyelonephritis (kidney
  infections)
renal – colic, cyst
urethra abnormalities
urethritis (infection of urethra)
urinary tract infections

RESPIRATORY

asbestosis
asthma
bronchitis
bronchiectasis (collapse of parts
  of lung tissue)
bronchospasm (wheezing)
emphysema
hay fever
laryngitis
larynx – polyps
lung – cystic fibrosis, embolism
  (clots), fibrosis

pleurisy
pneumonia
respiratory failure
respiratory tract infections
rhinorrhea (runny nose)
silicosis
Singer's nodes
sinusitis
status asthmaticus
tonsilitis
tracheitis (infection, allergies)
tuberculosis (TB)

SKELETO-MUSCULAR

achondroplasia (dwarfism)
anklosing spondylitis (curvature
  of spine)
arthritis
calcification – muscles
chondromalacia patella
  (softening of kneecap)
Dupuytron's contraction of fingers
exostoses (bony spurs)
fibrositis
fragilitas ossium (osteitis imperfecta
  – brittle bone disease)
ganglions (in rheumatoid arthritis)
gout
kyphosis (severe spinal curvature)
macrocephaly (enlarged head)
Marfan's Syndrome
Milroy's disease (very large legs)
myasthenia gravis
muscular dystrophy – Becker
  type, Duchenne's type
myopathy (weakness of muscles)
neck – spasmodic torticollis
  (spasms), stiff
neuroma (tumor on nerve)
osteoarthritis
osteogenesis imperfecta (brittle
  bone disease)

osteomalacia (bone softening)
osteomyelitis
osteoporosis (bone softening)
otosclerosis (arthritis of bones in ear)
polymyositis (muscle aches)
Reiter's Syndrome (arthritis with conjunctivitis)
rheumatism
rheumatoid arthritis
rickets causing dwarfism
sarcoidosis (inflammation of lungs)
scleroderma (thickening of tissues of hands and esophagus)
scoliosis (curvature of spine)
Sjogren's Syndrome (dry eyes, dry mouth)
spina bifida
supraspinatus tendonitis (frozen shoulder)
tennis elbow
tenosynovitis
vitamin D deficiency (rickets)

SKIN DISORDERS

acne
baldness
blackheads
blisters
boils
carbuncles
cellulitis (infected skin)
chilblains
cold urticaria (hives from cold water)
dandruff (seborrheic dermatitis)
Dercum's disease (many fatty cysts)
dermatitis
ectropion (drooping lower eyelid)
eczema
fat tumor (lipoma)
icthyosis (severe scaling of skin)
impetigo
keloid (increased scar tissue)
livedo reticularis (as occurs in SLE: purple network of veins)
lupus erythematosus disseminated (SLE)
moles – benign, malignant
molluscum contagiousum (warts)
neurodermatitis
nevus (birth mark)
pellagra (low Vitamin B_3, niacin)
photodermatitis (from sunlight)
pityriasis – alba (white blotches on face)
port-wine hemangioma
psoriasis (flaky skin)
pustule (pimples)
rodent ulcer (skin cancer)
rosasea (bright red face)
scurvy (low Vitamin C)
sebaceous cysts
warts – oral, plantar, venereal
xeroderma pigmentosum (scaly skin and light sensitivity)

APPENDIX B

SYMPTOMS AND SIGNS

abdominal pain
achalasia (difficulty swallowing)
aging (premature)
alopecia (baldness)
angina
anhedonia (loss of interest in
    things)
ankle swelling,
anorexia (loss of appetite)
apathy
arachnodactyly (long fingers)
arcus senilis (white line around
    iris)
arrhythmias (irregular heart beat)
ataxia (staggering)
autism
back pain
balance disturbance
bedwetting (enuresis)
blindness
blood pressure – low
blue fingers, hands, sclera
    (whites of eyes), skin
blurred vision
blushing
bow legs
bradycardia (slow heart beat)
breathless (dyspnea)
brittle – bones, nails
bruising
buffalo hump
butterfly rash on face
chest deformities
chest pain
clubbing of fingers
colic
coma
constipation

convulsions/fits/turns
coordination – poor
cough
cracks in corners of mouth
cramps
dandruff
deafness
delerium
depressions
diarrhea
dizziness (vertigo)
drowsiness
dysmenorrhea (period pains)
dyspepsia (indigestion)
earache
energy low (neurasthenia)
epistaxis (nose bleeds)
excessive thirst
exhaustion
exophthalmos (protruding eyes)
eyebrows – bushy, droopy
fainting attacks
fatigue
fears
fever
fissured tongue
fits
flatulence
flushed
frequency – bowel, urine
frigidity
furred tongue
gangrene
geographic tongue (cracks in
    tongue)
giddiness
glossitis (shiny tongue)
grandiose delusions

271

growth retardation
guilt
gum bleeding
habit spasms (twitching)
hematemesis (vomits blood)
hemiplegia (strokes down one side)
hemoptysis (coughing up blood)
hemorrhage
hair kinky
hairiness
halitosis (bad breath)
headaches
heartburn
hiccups
hirsutism (hair on upper lip of women)
hoarseness
hyperactivity
hyperacusis (acutely aware of sounds)
impotence
impulsiveness
incontinence
infertility
insanity
insomnia
intentional tremor (mild shaking)
itching
jaundice
judgment – impaired
koilonychia (flat fingernails)
lassitude
lumbago
melancholia
migraine
mood swings
mouth breathing, dryness, ulcers
muscle atrophy – cramps, spasms, weakness
muscle wasting
myalgia (muscle aches)
myositis (muscle inflammation)

nails – biting, brittle, spooning, white dots
neurasthenia (lack of energy)
neuritis (inflammation of nerves)
night blindness
nightmares and night terrors
nocturnal muscle cramp
nose bleeding
numbness
nystagmus (eye flickers)
obsessions
orgasm – lack of
pain – back, bone, cardiac, chest, gall bladder, kidney stone, menstrual, muscle, urinary, bladder
pallor
palms – yellow
palpitation
paresthesia (pins and needles)
peeling of lips
persecutory delusions
photophobia (sensitivity to light)
photosensitivity (burns easily in sun)
pigmentation (unusual coloring)
postural abnormalities
pot belly
ptosis (droopy eyelids)
puberty – precocious
rashes
restlessness
retching (dry vomiting)
ringing in ears
sacro-iliitis (low back pains)
sciatica
senility
shock
shoulder pain
skin – blisters, café-au-lait spots, moles, ulcers, vitiligo (white spots), warts
skull thickening

sleep disturbances – insomnia,
night terrors, nightmares,
walking
slurred speech
sneezing
spasmodic torticollis (twisted
neck)
speech abnormalities
spine – backache
squint
stiff neck
sweating abnormalities –
excessive
swelling of feet
tachycardia (rapid heart beat)
taste abnormalities
tetany
thirst – excessive
thought disorder
throat – sore
tic
tiredness
tongue soreness
tremor
urination disturbances
vision – double
vomiting
weakness
weight – gain, loss
wheeze
wrist problems
xanthelasma (yellowish-pink
fatty plaques on eyelids)

PSYCHIATRIC
SYMPTOMS/PROBLEMS

addiction (alcohol, barbiturates,
analgesics, heroin, coffee,
cigarettes, etc.)
aggression
alcoholism
anorexia nervosa
antisocial behavior
anxiety state

appetite poor
autism
bad habits (nail biting, thumb
sucking, etc.)
behavioral disorders
blackouts
catatonia (statue-like state)
compulsions
concentration – poor
confusion
convulsions/fits/turns
coordination – poor
delinquency
delusions – grandiose
dementia
depersonalization (feel strange,
unreal)
depressions
derealization (surroundings
appear strange, unreal)
dirt eating (pica)
dizziness
dyskinesia (uncontrollable
movements)
dysmenorrhea (pain with
menstruation)
dyspepsia (indigestion)
ejaculation, premature
epilepsy
exhibitionism
fainting attacks
fearful
frigidity
guilt complex
habit spasms
hallucinations (imaginary sights
and sounds)
headaches
hyperactivity
hysterical
impotence
incontinence
insanity
insomnia
judgment – impaired

lassitude
libido (low)
mania (excessive activity)
manic-depressive psychosis
  (marked mood swings)
melancholia
memory defect in dementia
migraine
narcolepsy (irritable need to sleep)
nausea
nervousness
neurasthenia (chronic lack of
  energy)
neurodermatitis
neurosis
obsessional-compulsive neurosis
olfactory hallucinations
  (hallucinations of imaginary
  odors/smells)
panic attacks
paranoid delusions (persecutory
  or grandiose)

phobia
prefrontal leucotomy (psychosurgery)
presenile dementia
psychopath
psychosis
puerperal psychosis (postnatal)
reading disorders
restlessness
rituals
schizophrenia
school refusal syndrome
seizures
senile dementia
sexual – impotence, orgasm
  lack, precocity
suicide – attempt, behavior
tension
thought disorder
violence
war neurosis

APPENDIX C

CONGENITAL DEFECTS

cleft – lip, palate

club foot

coarctation of aorta (narrowing or aorta)

colobomata (defect in iris)

dwarfism

feet deformity – talipes (club foot)

hare-lip

heart defects

heart murmurs

hypospadius (malformed urethra)

imperforate anus (anus unopened at birth)

maldescended testis

meningocele (spinal cord uncovered)

nevus (mole/birth mark)

pectus – carinatum (pigeon chest), excavatum (shrunken chest)

polydactyly (extra finger)

pyloric stenosis (narrowing of stomach opening)

spine – congenital abnormalities

Sturge-Weber Syndrome (port-wine birth mark on face and
    calcification of brain)

syndactyly of fingers (webbed)

testis ectopic (testis in abnormal position)

tongue – angioma (blood vessel tumor on the tongue)

trisomy 21 syndrome: Down's Syndrome and heart defects

Turner's Syndrome (webbed neck, coarctation of aorta, short stature)

ureter double

uterine – congenital malformations

APPENDIX D

Phenotype/physical characteristics

SHORT STATURE

Achondroplasia (normal head and trunk size but short arms and legs)

Dwarfism (short limbs and trunk)

Stunted growth/pot belly (celiac disease/allergy to wheat/grains)

Progeria (severe premature aging and very short stature)

Werner's Syndrome (premature aging and short stature)

TALL STATURE

Gigantism/Acromegaly (enlarged hands, feet, skull, etc.)

Klinefelter's Syndrome (tall but small testes) (XXY)

Marfan's Syndrome (arachnodactyly: slim with long, thin fingers, lens changes in eyes, ectopia lentils)

Homocystinuria (similar to above)

FAT/OBESE

Hypothyroidism (underactive thyroid) with coarse facial features, loss of hair, loss of outer third of eyebrows, hoarse voice, poor coordination

Cushing's Syndrome (overactive adrenal cortex with raised cortisol) moon face, buffalo hump at base of neck, purple stretch marks (striae), bruising, thin/brittle skin, hair on face (hirsutes)

Dercum's disease – obese with multiple lipoma (fatty cysts)

Diabetes – leg ulcers, fatty plaques around the eyes (xanthelasma), caratacts/poor vision, leg amputated for gangrene or arterial occlusion, poor wound healing, prone to boils/infections, etc.

THIN (WITH ARTHRITIS)

SLE – prematurely gray hair, hair loss/alopecia, butterfly rash on face, blue hands when cold (Raynaud's phenomenon), rashes, mouth ulcers, lassitude, weakness, depression or psychoses. Pernicious anemia is sometimes present.

THIN WITH AGITATION/ ANXIETY STATE

Hyperthyroidism (overactive thyroid) – protruding eyes (exophthalmos), increased sweating, reddish palms, racing pulse, impaired eye movements, weakness, depression or psychosis.

276

APPENDIX E

Sociological/epidemiological data

AGE
SEX
DATE OF BIRTH
DATE/AGE AT DEATH
PLACE OF BIRTH
- city
- country
- inland
- near the sea
- near pine forest, etc.
- drank tap, bore or tank water (from rain water run-off) during pregnancy/as a child
RACE: (e.g., Caucasian)
RELIGION: (e.g., Seventh Day Adventist, avoids meats)
MARITAL STATUS:
EDUCATION/QUALIFICATIONS:
OCCUPATION/PROFESSION:
DEPRIVED/UNDERPRIVILIGED or not during childhood, pregnancy
DIET: vegetarian or not
HABITS: cigarettes/tobacco (daily amount), alcohol (amount, type), barbiturates, analgesics, others
PETS: dogs, cats, birds, mice, rabbits, horses, goats
LIVED ON A FARM WITH ANIMALS:
SPORTING ACTIVITIES: jogging, cricket, golf, swimming, etc.
CREATIVE INTERESTS: music/composing, writing/poetry, public speaking/debating, art/painting, sculpture, photography, dancing/ballet
HISTORICAL FACTS OF INTEREST:
FAMOUS: sportsman, excellent in exams, artist, politician, public speaker, clergyman, doctor, actor, singer, musician/composer, architect, lawyer, inventor, astronaut

CLAIM TO FAME: records in sport; first to discover: new disease, new scientific facts, climb mountain, lived to 100 (record diet/habits/interests/secret of longevity)

BLACK SHEEP OF FAMILY (could indicate missed illnesses): trouble at school, truancy, expelled from school, trouble with police, stealing, shoplifting, spent time in jail, trouble with law, fraud, murder, assaults

PERSONALITY DISTURBANCE: dependent, sociopathic (psychopathic/ antisocial), hysterical, inadequate, schizoid, paranoid, obsessional/ compulsive, passive/aggressive

APPENDIX F

Questionnaire

Has anyone had the following:

1. CANCER:

In particular bowel, gastric (stomach), breast, uterine (womb), esophagus, leukemia, melanoma, lung, skin, brain tumor, liver, pancreas, lymphoma, Hodgkin's disease.

2. ENDOCRINE/GLANDULAR DISORDERS AND AUTOIMMUNE DISEASE:

[i] (a) Diabetes, (history of boils, cataracts, gangrene, on insulin or special diet and women who give birth to babies over nine pounds); (b) pancreatitis; (c) cystic fibrosis.

[ii] **Thyroid disorder:** (a) overactive thyroid – thin, agitated, marked stare, racing pulse, diarrhea; (b) underactive thyroid – overweight, sluggish/slowed down, poor recent memory, voice becoming hoarse, aches/pains in wrists, going deaf, yellowish complexion, losing hair, hypertension; (c) thyroid dysfunction – goiter, Hashimoto's disease, thyroid cysts.

[iii] **Pernicious anemia:** the signs include broad forehead, blue/gray eyes, gray hair before 40, vitiligo/leucoderma (white depigmented areas on legs and arms), shiny red tongue, diarrhea, depressed/confused/psychotic, history of anemia needing B_{12} or raw liver, tingling sensation (paraesthesia) in hands and feet, even paralysis.

[iv] **Cushing's Syndrome** (overactive adrenal cortex with raised cortisol); overweight, purple striae (stretch marks), buffalo hump back of neck between shoulders, moon face, bruises easily, depressed, psychotic, hypomanic (talks excessively). Hirsutes (hair on upper lip and chin) usually present.

[v] Addison's disease (underactive adrenal cortex with low cortisol): increased skin pigmentation, low blood pressure, weak, depressed, psychotic, thin, prone to infections especially "thrush" (monilia/*candida albicans*).

[vi] Parathyroid glands: (a) overactive (hyperparathyroidism) with raised calcium and kidney stones (usually recurrent), bone disorder, weakness/wasting of muscles, depression or psychosis, abdominal pain/duodenal ulcers; (b) underactive (hypoparathyroidism) with low blood calcium and tendency to cramps, weakness, tetany or fits, psychosis, depression and tendency to soft tissue calcification.

[vii] Thymus: tumor of the thymus/thymoma may result in myasthenia gravis (in 10 percent of cases) with severe lassitude and weakness. Droopy eyelids (ptosis) and double vision are common and also smooth fairly immobile facial features.

[viii] Disorder of ovaries: (a) Hypofunction – delayed menarche (breast development, skeletal growth, appearance of pubic hair, etc.), early menopause (hot flushes), osteoporosis (bones become brittle), dyspareunia (painful intercourse) and depression; (b) Hyperfunction may cause (i) feminizing tumors with pseudo precocious puberty/menstruation at an early age; (ii) masculinizing tumors; (iii) precocious puberty due to pituitary gland over stimulation of the ovaries; (iv) Stein-Leventhal Syndrome with hirsutes (hair on upper lip and chin), polycystic ovaries, irregular menstrual cycles often with long period of amenorrhea (no menstruation) and abnormal bleeding, +/- virilism (masculinization).

[ix] Disorders of testes: (a) Hypofunction – delayed puberty may be due to underactive pituitary, thyroid or testicular disease; (b) Hyperfunction – tumor of testes with precocious puberty/sexual development before ten years of age.

[x] Pituitary dysfunction: (a) Hypopituitarism (underactive pituitary) with weakness, lassitude, headaches, cold intolerance, disturbed sexual function, short stature and underdevelopment of sexual organs. Adults lack axillary and pubic hair, have genital and breast underdevelopment, pale skin and nipples, wrinkled face, poor muscle development and appear prematurely aged; (b) Hyperpituitarism (i) growth hormone is released in excess resulting in acromegaly/gigantism (ii) prolactin excess resulting in galactorrhea (breast releasing milk)/amenorrhea (cessation of menstruation) (iii) ACTH in excess resulting in Cushing's Syndrome (see 2[iv]).

[xi] Other rarer tumors/glandular/endocrine disorders include: (a) Adrenal cortex tumor (Conn's Syndrome) – excessive aldosterone hormone production with hypertension (high blood pressure), excessive loss of potassium and retention of sodium, hence weakness/lassitude and complaints of headaches; (b) Adrenal medulla tumor (central part of adrenal gland), such as phaeochromocytoma, with marked sweating, palpitations, nervousness, tremor, weight loss, pallor and flushing, heat intolerance and with tendency to high blood pressure (or low blood pressure); (c) Carcinoid Syndrome – tumor of stomach or gut – flushed skin of head and neck mainly, diarrhea, wheezing, heart problems and racing pulse or high blood pressure; (d) Diabetes insipidus – excessive thirst, polydipsia (high intake of water) and polyuria (excessive amounts of water passed); (e) Ectopic hormone production – many tumors can secrete hormones especially lung, thyroid, adrenal, ovarian, breast, pancreatic, skin/melanoma, kidney, liver, stomach and bowel cancers; (f) Pancreatic tumors – (i) Zollinger-Ellison – releasing gastrin with severe peptic (stomach/duodenal) ulcers; (ii) Insulinoma – resulting in hypoglycemia (low blood sugar); (iii) Glucagonoma – resulting in raised blood sugar, dermatitis, weight loss, anemia; (iv) Somatostatin – resulting in diarrhea and anemia; (g) Pineal tumors – precocious puberty or depressed sexual function, sometimes paralysis or upward gaze.

3. Arthritic conditions

Gout – very sore thumb/elbow or big toe, knees, etc. with raised uric acid made worse by too much fish/seafood (especially oysters, caviar), rhubarb, spinach, strawberries, alcohol and certain drugs. History of needing Xyloprim, Allopurinol or Colchicine suggests gout. Tophi (chalky outgrowth) can occur on the ears and elbows.

SLE (systemic lupus erythematosus) – arthritis with migrainous headaches, hair loss, rashes, mouth ulcers, photosensitivity (burns easily in the sun especially if butterfly shaped red rash

appears on the face), blue hands when cold (Raynaud's phenomenon) and allergy/intolerance to penicillin, sulphonamides, contraceptive pill, estrogens. Depression, confusion, psychosis,
severe lassitude, weakness and proneness to lung and bladder
infections are very common. Often the whole body aches.
Allergies to grains (gluten), eggs, milk, yeast, beef and/or
legumes are extremely common and the condition will usually
remit when these are omitted from the diet. Lung, heart, liver
and kidney can also be severely involved. Usually treated with
steroids/prednisone.

Rheumatoid arthritis – deforming arthritis of hands and joints
usually made worse by citrus (oranges, etc.) and solanaceae
(tobacco, tomato, eggplant, capsicum, pepper, potato, paprika,
etc.). History of treatment with asprin/salicylates, naprosyn,
indocid, gold therapy, etc. Allergies to dairy products/grains are
usually associated.

**Juvenile rheumatoid arthritis (JRA) (a) Systemic (25 percent
of JRA)** – usually starts in males aged five. They have fever,
rashes, heart involvement such as pericarditis (lining of the
heart is inflamed), myocarditis (muscle of heart is inflamed).
Lungs may be affected (pneumonitis, pleurisy) and cases
often go on to severe joint involvement (Still's disease).
(b) Pauciarticular arthritis (30 percent of JRA) – a mild form of
arthritis of the knees and ankles which usually affects females
from two to four years of age. About half the patients may
have eye involvement which can develop into cataracts.
(c) Polyarticular arthritis (25 percent of JRA) – in girls mainly,
about two years of age. Slowly affects joints of hands and feet.

Osteoarthritis – affecting big joints such as knees, hips, as well
as feet, hands, back/neck. Joints in the hands have hard
swellings on the side of fingers (Heberden's nodes).
Immunology suggests allergy/intolerance/hypersensitivity to
toxic factions of wheat and other grains containing gluten such
as rye, oats, barley, millet and buckwheat; food allergies to
those are usually present.

Ankylosing spondylitis – chronic progressive disease involv-
ing the spine and adjacent soft tissues. Sacroiliac joints are

always affected (middle of back at hip level). It usually accompanies blood group HLA: 27 and affects males in their thirties.

Sjogren's Syndrome – arthritis with dry eyes, dry mouth. Usually middle-aged women (only 10 percent are men). Lack of secretion may also affect lungs, stomach, skin and vagina.

Other arthritic conditions: (a) Arthritis with psoriasis (severe flaky skin condition). (b) Arthritis with ulcerative colitis (usually diarrhea and milk allergy/intolerance), usually affects the hands and feet (75 percent of patients) and in 25 percent spondylitis affects the back. (c) Arthritis with Crohn's disease – diarrhea and fissures in anal area. Arthritis affects mainly knees, hands and back. (d) Arthritis with urethritis (inflammation of the urethra/tube in the penis), conjunctivitis (inflammation of cornea or eye) and mouth ulcers (Reiter's Syndrome). (e) Behcet's Syndrome – recurrent ulcers of the mouth and genitalia together with eye inflammation and arthritis. (f) Whipple disease (intestinal lipodystrophy) – arthritis of the hands, feet, knees and ankles, together with weight loss, diarrhea, malabsorption of vitamins and minerals, and swollen glands. (g) Polyarteritis nodosa – arthritis with fever, weakness, loss of appetite, muscle aches, abdominal pain and sometimes severely impaired vision. There is inflammation of medium and small veins. (h) Giant-cell arteritis – can affect the temporal vessels and the patient complains of polymyalgia syndrome (aching pain and stiffness in the neck and shoulders, and pain in the lips and throat). (i) Progressive systemic sclerosis – involves fibrosis (thickening) of the skin (scleroderma) and internal organs such as esophagus, lungs, heart and kidney. The skin on the hands is tight and firm. Fingers are swollen and stiff. Hands tend to be blue in cold weather (Raynaud's phenomenon). There is pain in the fingers and joints and difficulty in swallowing. (j) Shoulder-hand syndrome – stiffness and weakness present. (k) Fibrositis – localized aches and tenderness in muscles. (l) Carpal tunnel syndrome – numbness and burning pain in the hand and wrist made worse by movement. (m) Relapsing polychondritis – inflammation and destruction of cartilage especially of nose and ears. Fever and arthritis are commonly associated. (n) Tietze's Syndrome – swelling, pain and tenderness where the ribs and sternum join. (o) Bursitis –

inflammation of the pockets of fluid between tendons, muscles and bony prominences, especially at the shoulder. (p) Tenosynovitis – inflammation of the synovial lining of tendons.

4 BLOOD DISORDERS:

Anemia (low hemoglobin) record cause if known, such as due to iron deficiency, low Vitamin B_{12} (pernicious anemia), hemolytic (where red cells are breaking down), low folic acid, etc.

Leukemia – type where known, such as Hodgkin's disease.

Bleeding/clotting disorder – hemophilia, platelet disorders, other conditions where known.

Polycythemia – raised hemoglobin with tendency to thrombosis, headaches, dizziness, depression, confusion and spots before the eyes.

5. RESPIRATORY DISORDERS:

Asthma, pneumonia, pleurisy, atalectasis (collapsed lung especially in premature-birth children), emphysema (chronic obstructive airways disease), TB, fibrosis of the lung, silicosis, asbestosis, abscess, fungal infections, embolism (blood clot in the lung vessels).

6. GASTROINTESTINAL DISORDERS:

Shiny tongue, furred tongue, sore tongue, mouth ulcers, fissured tongue, cracked lips, esophagitis (inflammation of esophagus), hiatus hernia, reflux esophatitis/water brash, stomach (gastric) ulcer, stomach cancer, esophageal varices (veins swollen), pyloric stenosis (narrowing of opening leading from stomach to pylorus), duodenal ulcer, Crohn's disease (regional ileitis), intussesception (telescoping of ileum into cecum), dysentery, appendicitis, diverticulitis, diverticulosis, cancer of colon, mesenteric adenitis (swollen glands in the abdomen), bowel cancer, rectal cancer, anal fissure, hemorrhoids.

Liver disorder – hepatitis, cirrhosis, gallstones, gall bladder inflammation (choleycystitis), cancer.

Pancreas disorders – pancreatitis, tumor, cystic fibrosis, diabetes.

7. Epilepsy:

Record type such as grand mal, petit mal, temporal lobe (psychomotor), gelastic, febrile convulsions, hypsarrythmia, idiopathic (cause unknown), post traumatic (head injury), blackouts.

8. Disorders of central nervous system:

Headaches, migraine, epilepsy, meningitis, encephalitis, brain tumors, brain abscess, cerebellar tumor, cerebrovascular accident – hemorrhage or thrombosis (stroke), Parkinson's disease, hardening of arteries (arteriosclerosis), senility (Alzheimer's disease), pellagra/low Vitamin B_3, pernicious anemia/low Vitamin B_{12}, hypothyroidism/underactive thyroid, low Vitamin B_1, low zinc, SLE (systemic lupus erythematosus), multiple sclerosis, motor neuron disease/amyotrophic lateral sclerosis, trigemial neuralgia (severe facial pain/tic douloureux), Bell's palsy (facial nerve palsy/drooping of side of face/mouth), optic neuritis (inflammation of optic nerve), nystagmus (jerking movement of the eyes), neurosyphilis/GPI (general paralysis of the insane).

9. Skin disorders:

Seborrheic dermatitis/dandruff, psoriasis, urticaria, hives, cellulitis, infantile eczema, eczema, scurvy, dry skin, skin cancers, moles/melanoma, angular cheilosis/stomatitis – cracks at corner of mouth (low Vitamin B_2, etc), vitiligo/leucoderma – white depigmented areas in the skin, dark pigmented areas, warts, pityriasis alba – round areas of fine depigmentation on the face, hands or trunk, ecchymoses – areas of bruising (usually due to low Vitamin C), tinnea – capitis (head) – cruris (groin), monilia/thrush/*candida albicans*, varicose veins and varicose vein ulcers, shingles (Herpes zoster), boils (carbuncles), acne, blackheads (comedones), hordeola (stys), rashes (chicken pox, measles, etc.), blisters (allergic conditions, porphyria cutanea tarda).

(a) Nails (i) white dots – low in Vitamin B_6 and zinc. Often associated with pyroluria (positive Kryptopyrrole in the urine);

(ii) flat nails/cupped nails (Koilonychia/spooning) due to iron deficiency and malabsorption states; (iii) clubbed nails – lung disorders and cystic fibrosis; (iv) pitting of nails – psoriasis; (v) onycholysis (lifting nails) – overactive thyroid; (vi) brittle/chalky nails – low calcium and magnesium; (vii) infection at side of nail (paronychia) – fungal infection; (viii) white nails – liver disorder.

10. GENITOURINARY SYSTEM:

(Kidney, ureter, bladder, prostate, urethra): kidney stones, kidney/bladder infections, glomerulonephritis/Bright's disease, kidney failure, renal colic, one kidney, horse-shoe kidney, bladder tumor, bladder stones, trigonitis (inflammation of trigone area due to virus/allergy with urgency/frequency), nocturia (need to pass water at night), dysuria (pain on passing urine), prostate hypertrophy (enlargement), prostatitis (inflammation of prostate), prostatic cancer, urethritis (painful urethra due to inflammation/infection), balinitis (infection under foreskin), herpes simplex, syphilis or other venereal disease.

11. INFECTION:

Tuberculosis, glandular fever (infectious mononucleosis), mumps, measles, scarlet fever, chicken pox, influenza, rheumatic fever, viral diphtheria, meningitis, encephalitis, hepatitis viral A (infectious) and viral B (serum) – seen in drug addicts, whooping cough, dysentery, cholera, amebiasis, malaria, Dengue fever, scrub typhus, hydatids, fungal infections (monilia/thrush/*candida albicans*, etc.), giardia lamblia, trichomonas, others.

12. PSYCHIATRIC DISORDERS:

Depressive illness, mood swings (manic-depressive illness), psychoses, schizophrenia, senile dementia/confusion, chronic lassitude/neurasthenia, personality disorders (obsessional/compulsive, paranoid, schizoid, hysterical, sociopathic/psychopathic, inadequate, dependent, passive-aggressive), addiction (alcohol, barbiturates, heroin opiates, caffeine, others).

13. CHILDHOOD DISORDERS:

Autism, hyperactivity, behavior disorders, learning disorders, temper tantrums, head banging, thumb sucking, enuresis (bed wetting), encopresis (soiling underclothes), school phobia/

truancy, epilepsy, delayed bone growth, delayed motor development, sleep disorders, night phobia, night terrors, nightmares, sleep walking (somnambulism).

14. Muscle disorders:

Myasthenia gravis, muscular dystrophy, myotonia dystrophica, myositis [i] viral [ii] allergic, motor neuron disease (amyotrophic lateral sclerosis), poliomyelitis, polymyositis, ME (myalgic encephalamyelitis).

15. Gynecological:

Big babies (over 4 kg, mother at risk for diabetes later), breast cysts/lumps/cancer, eclampsia (fit in pregnancy), ectopic pregnancy, endometriosis (chocolate cysts), fibroids, hysterectomy, mastitis (inflammation of breast), menorrhagia (heavy periods), miscarriage, polycystic ovaries, cravings in pregnancy, postnatal or puerperal depression/psychosis, vaginitis, womb (uterine) cancer.

16. Allergies:

(a) **Drugs** – barbiturates, penicillin, sulphonamides, opiates, anaesthetics, contraceptive pill, estrogens, others.

(b) **Food** – grains/wheat, milk, eggs, yeast, beef.

(c) **Inhalant allergies** – house dust, house mites, tree and grass pollens, hair of dogs, cats or cattle, hen feathers, molds, tobacco, smoke, wool, kapok, cotton.

(d) **Petrochemicals/chemicals/metals** – gasoline, fumes, soaps, perfumes, metals, sprays, etc.

(e) **Undiagnosed allergies:** have recognizable symptoms and signs including evidence of vitamin-mineral deficiencies. (a) Signs/symptoms of food/inhalant allergies. Puffy eyes, face, nose, shrunken eyes, dark area under eyes (allergic shiners), runny eyes, runny nose, urticaria (hives), flushed appearance, itchy/dry skin, sinusitis/headaches, glare intolerance, sore throat, indigestion, bloating, wind, diarrhea, constipation, halitosis (bad breath), abdominal pains, depressions, anxiety state, chronic lassitude, irritability, poor memory/concentration, psychosis and other psychiatric conditions/childhood disorders, muscle aches/pains and certain arthritis conditions. Associated are evidence of malabsorption state for vitamins/minerals. (ii) Evidence of vitamin-mineral deficiencies.

Low Vitamin B₁ (thiamine) – poor memory/concentration/ coordination, depression, irritability, agoraphobia, insomnia, abdominal pains, beri beri, Wernicke's encephalopathy, Korsakov's psychosis, foot drop, optic atrophy, anemia with large cells.

Low Vitamin B₂ (riboflavin) – cracks at corner of mouth, cracked lips, dry skin, dandruff, prone to conjunctivitis, infections, depression.

Low Vitamin B₃ (niacin) – fissured tongue, diarrhea, dermatitis, dementia, depression, psychosis/schizophrenia, behavior/ learning disorders, pellagra.

Low Vitamin B₅ (pantothenic acid) – depression, constipation, underactive adrenal gland, prone to infections.

Low Vitamin B₆ (pyridoxal) – depression, hyperactivity, epilep- sy, sleep disorders (no dreams, or if dreams then poor dream recall), white dots in nails (also associated with low zinc), tendency to thrombosis, tendency to anemia with small pale cells, also prone to infections.

Low Vitamin B₁₂ (pernicious anemia) – sore shiny red tongue, diarrhea, dementia, depression, psychosis, subacute degenera- tion of the cord, optic atrophy, heart failure, tendency to premature graying, lassitude, prone to infections.

Low folate (Vitamin Bc) – depression, confusion/dementia, psychosis, severe lassitude, neurological disorders, anemia with big red cells.

Low Vitamin E – poor muscle development/coordination, tendency to varicose veins/hemorrhoids, vascular (blood vessel) disorders, tendency to thrombosis, low libido, skin problems.

Low Vitamin C (ascorbic acid) – scurvy, bleeding gums, bruis- ing (capillary fragility), depression, psychosis, lassitude, low stress tolerance, prone to infections. Very important for con- nective tissue such as collagen and elastin and blood vessels/cartilage.

Low Vitamin A – glare intolerance, night blindness, dry skin, prone to infections/weak mucous membranes, cracked lips/tongue, sinusitis, important for adrenal cortex together with B_1, B_5 and Vitamin C.

Low Vitamin K – bleeding tendency with liver disorders.

Low Vitamin D – responsible for rickets, bow legs, caved in chest, bossing of forehead.

Low biotin – depression, poor testicular development.

Low zinc – white dots in nails, cracked lips, dry skin, glare intolerance, prone to infections, prone to creaking joints and cartilage problems, depression and lassitude. Tendency to have pyroluria (Kryptopyrrole in the urine with depression, headaches, lassitude, poor dream recall).

Low iron – can cause anemia or sideropaenia if hemoglobin not low, sore tongue, spooning or flat nails, depression, lassitude, learning/behavior problems, poor healing and tendency to infections.

Low calcium/magnesium – tendency to fits, muscle cramps, irritability, aching joints, poor teeth/bone development, depression, brittle/chalky nails and impaired immune system; important for heart and blood vessels and nervous system.

APPENDIX G

Keep smiling

Help for your mood, muscles, sanity,
memory, brain and to keep your hair on

ILLNESSES DUE TO NUTRIENT DEFICIENCIES

1. Nutrient deficiencies that can cause depression
2. Nutrient deficiencies that can cause lassitude/weakness
3. Nutrient deficiencies that can cause or aggravate psychosis
4. Nutrient deficiencies affecting memory and increasing risk for confusion and dementia
5. Nutrient deficiencies that can cause demyelination (breakdown of nerve myelin) and increase risk for paralysis
6. Nutrient deficiencies and conditions causing or aggravating hair loss (alopecia)

1. THE FOLLOWING NUTRIENT DEFICIENCIES CAN CAUSE DEPRESSION:

Vitamins

B_1 (Thiamine) beri beri
B_2 (Riboflavin)
B_3 (Niacin) pellagra
B_5 (Pantothenic acid)
B_6 (Pyridoxal)
B_{12} (Cobalamin) pernicious
    anaemia

Choline
Biotin
PABA
Inositol
C (Ascorbic acid) scurvy
Folic acid
E

Trace Elements

Sodium	Calcium	Zinc
Chloride	Phosphate	Iron
Potassium	Manganese	Selenium
Magnesium	Chromium	

Heavy Metals

Copper - can cause anemia and demyelination; also cofactor for SOD1 enzymes and brain metalloenzymes

Amino Acids
   L-tryptophan helps form
        – B_3 (Niacin)
        – Picolinic acid for optimal zinc absorption
        – Serotonin
        – Melatonin
        – PGE1 series (beneficial prostaglandins)
L-glutamine forms
        – γ GABA (gamma-aminobutyric acid)
DL-phenylalanine and L-tyrosine form
        – noradrenaline
        – adrenaline
        – tyramine
        – dopamine
L-glycine

2. THE FOLLOWING NUTRIENT DEFICIENCIES CAN CAUSE LASSITUDE/WEAKNESS:

Vitamins

B_1	B_6	Inositol
B_2	B_{12}	C
B_3	Biotin	Folic acid
B_5	PABA	E

Trace Elements

Sodium	Calcium	Zinc
Chloride	Phosphate	Iron
Potassium	Manganese	Selenium
Magnesium	Chromium	Germanium

Heavy Metals
   Copper

Essential Fatty Acids
   W3 EFAs
   W6 EFAs

Amino Acids
   Glutamine (contraindicated in hyperammonemia)
   In fact, most essential amino acids, if low, can affect energy.
   Amino acids are essential for muscle protein, etc.

CoQ10 (Ubiquinone/Co-enzyme Q10)

3. NUTRIENT DEFICIENCIES THAT CAN CAUSE OR AGGRAVATE PSYCHOSIS:

Vitamins

B_1	B_6	Vitamin C
B_3	B_{12}	Folic acid
B_5	Biotin	

Trace Elements

Potassium	Phosphate	Iron
Magnesium	Manganese	
Calcium	Zinc	

Heavy Metals
Copper

4. NUTRIENT DEFICIENCIES AFFECTING MEMORY AND INCREASING RISK FOR CONFUSION AND DEMENTIA:

Vitamins

B_1 (beri beri, Korsakoff's psychosis and Wernicke's encephalopathy)

B_3 (pellagra)

B_5 and Choline to form acetylcholine for cholinergic pathways, which are the first to break down in Alzheimer's disease.

B_6

B_{12} (pernicious anemia, subacute combined degeneration of the spinal cord)

Folic acid

Trace Elements

Sodium	Iron
Chloride	Magnesium
Potassium	Manganese } cofactors for B_1
Calcium	Zinc and B_6 to work
Phosphate	

Heavy Metals
Copper

Amino Acids
L-tryptophan (to form B_3)
Glutamine
Cysteine

Note: Most amino acids are essential for brain development and for brain maintenance.

5. Nutrient deficiencies that can cause or aggravate demyelination:

Vitamins

B_1	B_3	B_{12}
B_2	B_6	Folic acid

Trace Elements

Magnesium
Manganese ⎤ cofactors for B_1 and B_6 to work
Zinc ⎦

Heavy Metals

Copper – important for myelin and brain metalloenzymes, etc., and for SOD1 enzymes to detoxify free radicals

Note. My research shows many patients with MS and ALS are very low in B_1, B_3 and B_6. Some patients with pellagra (low B_3/niacin) can still be low in B_3 as measured when on 1800 mg of niacinamide daily. It follows, then, that patients with ALS need at least 2 grams (2000 mg) of B_3 to make sure they are not still low in B_3. As with ALS, low B_3 can cause bulbar palsy (paralysis of swallowing, talking and breathing) as well as paralysis of limbs, etc.

ALS = Amyotrophic Laterla Sclerosis or motor neuron disease
MS = Multiple Sclerosis

6. Conditions causing or aggravating hair loss (alopecia):

Vitamin deficiencies

B_{12} (Cobalt)	Biotin	PABA

Trace element deficiencies

Iron	Iodine + tyrosine to form T4
Cobalt (B_{12})	(thyroxine)
Zinc	

Hormone deficiencies

Cortisol
DHEA (dehydroepiandrosterone)
T4 (thyroxine)

Medical conditions

SLE (systemic lupus erythematosus)
Celiac disease (malabsorption for nutrients and damage to reticulin of hair follicles.)
Hypothyroidism (low T4, etc.)

APPENDIX H

Stay alive

Help for the vessels to your brain and heart.

A. Diagram of a blood vessel showing nutrients to protect the vessel wall.
   1. Endothelial lining
   2. Smooth muscle
   3. Fibrin
   4. Collagen
   5. Elastin
B. Diagnostic (pathology tests to discuss with your general practitioner or cardiologist.

   Tests to help prevent vasculitis or damage to vessel walls and hardening of arteries (arteriosclerosis) and risk for senility or heart attack or stroke or thrombosis (blood clot in brain or heart or lungs or leg, etc.).

A. DIAGRAMATIC CROSS SECTION OF A BLOOD VESSEL

All need B_1, B_3, B_6, Vitamin C, magnesium, zinc, manganese, copper, bioflavinoids, amino acids.

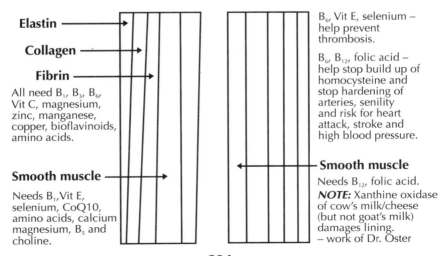

Elastin

Collagen

Fibrin

All need B_1, B_3, B_6, Vit C, magnesium, zinc, manganese, copper, bioflavinoids, amino acids.

Smooth muscle

Needs B_1, Vit E, selenium, CoQ10, amino acids, calcium magnesium, B_5 and choline.

B_6, Vit E, selenium – help prevent thrombosis.

B_6, B_{12}, folic acid – help stop build up of homocysteine and stop hardening of arteries, senility and risk for heart attack, stroke and high blood pressure.

Smooth muscle
Needs B_{12}, folic acid.
NOTE: Xanthine oxidase of cow's milk/cheese (but not goat's milk) damages lining.
– work of Dr. Öster

294

Endothelial lining antibodies positive – use the diet to help reverse synovitis.

Smooth muscle antibodies positive – use the diet to help reverse SLE.

Elastin antibodies positive – use the diet to help reverse synovitis.

Collagen antibodies positive – use the diet to help reverse synovitis.

Fibrin antibodies positive – use the diet to help reverse synovitis.

Diet to reverse SLE – see Appendix J
Diet to reverse synovitis – see Appendix K

B. DIAGNOSTIC (PATHOLOGY) TESTS TO DISCUSS WITH YOUR GENERAL PRACTITIONER OR CARDIOLOGIST.

1. Hemaglobin/film/ESR (sedimentation rate)

    a. Low hemaglobin – anemia

        i. if red cells are very small (low MCV/microcytosis) and very pale (low MCH), suspect low iron +/– low B_6/pyridoxal or Thalassemia (with raised fetal hemaglobin). The tests (on fasted blood) for low B_6 are (a) P-5-P; (b) EGOT and (c) EGOT + P-5-P and for iron are Iron Studies. **Low iron** is often seen with tear-shaped cells (poikilocytes) or target cells. **Raised iron** can be seen with hemachromatosis with raised serum iron, transferrin saturation and/or ferritin (iron stores) and also with risk for coronary artery disease and diabetes. Genetic testing looking at C282y and H63D mutation confirms diagnosis of hemachromotosis. Raised iron can occur with acute intermittent porphyria (King George III disease), especially if glucose also is raised.

       ii. if red cells are very big (high MCV/macrocytosis), then suspect low B_1, B_3, B_{12}, folic acid, Vitamin C, manganese, T4 (thyroxine – a thyroid hormone), alcohol (tippler) or medication side effects.

      iii. if red cells are smaller than average size (7.2 Angstrom), but MCV is not low and bigger than average, but not raised MCV, this is called "anisocytosis" and the anemia is called "normocytic" (not low or raised MCV, i.e., not microcytosis or macrocytosis as outlined above) and normochromic (normal color, not low or raised MCH as outlined above). This suggests low iron +/– B_6 are trying to make red cells smaller than usual and low B_1 or B_3 or B_{12} or Vitamin C or folic acid or manganese or T4 is trying to make red cells bigger than usual. Thus, the anemia can be due to combinations of these nutrient deficiencies.

   b. Raised hemaglobin – such conditions as polycythemia vera or secondary polycythemia with risk for thrombosis are likely.

   c. Raised ESR (sedimentation rate) – suspect infection, inflammation, arthritis, collagen/connective tissue disorder such as rheumatoid arthritis or SLE, risk for cancer or increased risk for thrombosis, etc.

There are numerous conditions associated with abnormal blood films and another useful test is live red cell examination – use "Dark Field Testing."

2. Fasting cholesterol and triglycerides

   a. Raised cholesterol and triglycerides increase the risk for heart attacks and strokes.

   b. Lipid EPG looks at levels of LDL (bad oil) and HDL (good oil) and helps to clarify the type of cholesterol or lipid disorder. The ratio of cholesterol/HDL gives the "CHD," i.e., risk for a heart attack, stroke, etc.

   c. Low cholesterol can increase the risk for thrombosis and coronary artery disease, heart attack and stroke, if associated with low serum DHEAS (dehydroepiandrosterone) hormone. Cholesterol is an essential precursor to form DHEAS. Cholesterol can be low in (i) celiac disease, which is associated with over a hundred other illnesses, including low serum DHEAS and low vitamins, minerals, amino acids, to protect the vessel lining and wall (see diagram of cross section of a vessel and associated nutrients for the vessel wall) and low levels of nutrients such as B_6, Vitamin E, selenium, increase risk for thrombosis; (ii) Tangier disease with low cholesterol and low HDL and low APO A1; (iii) hypobetalipoproteinemia with low cholesterol and low triglycerides and low APO B.

3. **Fasted levels of Vitamins B_6, E and selenium** help fight against thrombosis risk.

4. **Serum homocysteine** – if raised, there is an increased risk for hardening of arteries/senility and thrombosis/heart attack/stroke. A deficiency in Vitamins B_6, B_{12} and folic acid increase the risk for these developing. Homocysteinemia patients on Vitamin B_6 have far less thromboses.

5. **Fasted levels of Vitamin B_{12} and folic acid** – if low, would indicate the plasmologen lining of vessels is more likely to be impaired and the risk for varicose veins/ulcers is more likely. Good levels of B_{12} and folic acid help stop homocysteine build-up, causing hardening of arteries, thrombosis, etc.

6. **Serum DHEAS hormone** – when low, is associated with risk for many illnesses including coronary artery disease, stroke, heart attack, diabetes, senility, Alzheimer's disease, cancer, as well as many neurological conditions including MS (multiple sclerosis), ALS (motor neuron disease), cerebellar atrophy, Huntington's chorea, Parkinson's disease. Low DHEAS is also commonly seen with raised cholesterol (can't convert it to DHEAS – biotin may help).

7. **Lipoprotein a, i.e., LP(a)** – a raised level is seen with arterio-sclerosis (risk for hardening of arteries). This is a type of LDL – "bad oil."

8. **ANF** positive is seen with risk for different types of collagen/connective tissue disorder with risk for high blood pressure, heart attack, stroke and thrombosis. To exclude SLE (systemic lupus ery-thematosus) the following tests are useful – ANF and if positive then ds DNA; if this is raised, would confirm the condition. If not raised, then it would be wise to do ENA screen for SLE (or other ANF posi-tive conditions, including Sjogren's Syndrome, scleroderma, pol-yarteritis nodosa), and a positive result indicates SLE. Even without a positive result, it is still possible to have SLE, and the following should be checked before any change in diet – C3 or C4 comple-ments low in SLE; immune complexes raised in SLE; immunoglobu-lins IgA, IgM and IgG raised in SLE; anti-lymphocyte antibodies raised in SLE. If these are normal, the diagnosis is most likely not SLE, with ds DNA not raised and ENA screen negative as well.

    However, if they are abnormal or some are grossly abnormal, then a skin biopsy should be done on unexposed skin (inner side of upper arm suggested) with immunoflorescent technique. Normally, at the dermo/epidermal junction in the skin, it is clear with no deposits of gammaglobulins, etc. However, in SLE, there are linear deposits or bands or discrete granules (cytoid bodies) of IgM or IgG or IgA or C1q or C3 or fibrin, supporting the diagnosis of SLE.

9. **ANCA antibodies.** This can help detect serious vascular condi-tions (i.e., affecting blood vessels) causing high blood pressure, stroke risk such as temporal arteritis, polyarteritis nodosa, Wegener's granulamatosis, etc. A diet such as the one to help reverse synovitis, as in Appendix K, is wise.

10. **Smooth muscle antibodies.** Smooth muscle is involuntary mus-cle in vessels, organs, gut, liver, etc., and a proliferation of smooth muscle can cause hypertension (high blood pressure), etc. Positive antibodies can be seen in lupus hepatitis (SLE), etc., and these

antibodies can be reversed to negative on a specific diet (see Appendix J) and by killing off the opportunist pathogens/bacteria, chlamydia pneumonia living in vessels, etc.

11. **Chlamydia pneumonia titre.** This bacteria is associated with pneumonia, recurrent chest infections, pleurisy, asthma, pericarditis, cardiomyopathy, coronary artery disease, and is commonly seen also in MS (multiple sclerosis).

12. **Immunoglobulins IgA, IgM, IgG** – raised in SLE, etc. Raised gammaglobulins are called "dysproteinemias" and are associated with risk for thrombosis and especially with SLE. Usually an EPG (electrophoretogram) looking at different types of protein, is done to exclude abnormal levels of protein – "paraproteinemias" such as multiple myeloma, which is another risk factor for thrombosis.

13. **Thyroid function tests** to exclude an underactive thyroid with risk for thrombosis or an overactive thyroid with risk for atrial fibrillation (an arrythmia) and risk for heart failure.

14. **Fasted glucose.** Glucose is raised in diabetes and less often is raised in acute intermittent porphyria, especially if iron is raised as well.

15. **Tests for cancer** which can be associated with risk for thrombosis, such as certain tumor markers as CEA for breast, stomach, lung, bowel cancer.

16. **Other special tests** (done by very few laboratories) to help diagnose and prevent vasculitis (narrowing of vessel lumen/opening due to proliferation of endothelial lining or elastin or collagen or fibrin of vessel walls. Those tests would include:
    – Endothelial antibodies (antibodies to the inner lining of vessels)
    – Elastin antibodies
    – Collagen antibodies
    – Fibrin antibodies

These can be reversed or reduced by the diet that helps reverse synovitis (see Appendix K).

When a person has high cholesterol and triglycerides, all the following increase risk for coronary artery disease, heart attack, stroke, hypertension, etc.:
Microcytic anemia with low B_6 +/- low iron
Raised ESR
Low B_{12} with macrocytic anemia
Low folic acid with macrocytic anemia
Low B_1/thiamine with macrocytic anemia

Low Vitamin C with macrocytic anemia
Raised homocysteine (due to low B_6, B_{12}, folic acid)
Low selenium
Low Vitamin E
Low serum DHEAS
Raised LP(a)
ANF positive with raised ds DNA (SLE)
Raised ANCA antibodies
Raised smooth muscle antibodies
Raised chlamydia pneumonia titre
Raised immunoglobulins (dysproteinemia)
Raised TSH
Raised glucose
Raised elastin antibodies
Raised collagen antibodies
Raised fibrin antibodies
Raised endothelial antibodies

The more a person has of the above risk factors, the worse the prognosis, and the more the risk for premature death from coronary artery disease, heart attack, stroke, thrombosis, hypertension, etc.

APPENDIX I

Don't sieze up

Help for your joints and painful limbs

A. FOODS TO AVOID WITH OSTEOARTHRITIS OR TO HELP PREVENT IT

	GRAINS	DAIRY PRODUCTS	YEAST
	Wheat, rye, oats, corn (maize), malt/barley, millet, buckwheat, cane sugar/syrup, molasses, treacle, bamboo shoots and asparagus	Cow's milk, cream, cheese, ice cream, yogurt, custard, products containing casein/ cow's milk, beef, veal, ox tongue, buffalo, gelatin (bovine protein)	Baker's yeast, brewer's yeast, yeast fractions as in wine, vinegar, bread, mushrooms, walnuts, molds. Problems with yeast extracts
DAMAGING FRACTIONS	Gluten, α-gliadin and glycoproteins of gluten-containing grains and in sugar	Especially α-casein, α-lactalbumin, β-lactoglobulin and other peptides in cow's milk. Also beef albumin and globulin	Glycoprotein fractions of yeast, molds and virus capsules and candida, etc.

B. SAFER FOODS FOR OSTEOARTHRITIS
(OFF COW'S MILK, GLUTEN-CONTAINING GRAINS, ETC.)

GRAINS: Rice, sunflower seeds, pumpkin seeds, linseed (flaxseed), rice flakes, puffed rice, rice bran, rice cakes, rice biscuits, 100% rice bread, rice syrup, maple syrup (true), honey – red gum, yellow box, (forest flower), but not molasses honey.

MILK: Rice milk, coconut milk, sheep's milk, goat's milk preferably from goats that are not grain fed.

The above should be under medical supervision.

APPENDIX J

Don't let lupus get you

Help for Systemic Lupus Erythematosus sufferers

A. FOODS TO BE AVOIDED FOR DIETARY INTERVENTION IN SLE (SYSTEMIC LUPUS ERYTHEMATOSUS)

The following foods (and pollens, as far as possible) are best avoided for at least eighteen months – some indefinitely as symptoms of SLE keep returning when those foods are reintroduced.

	GRAINS Wheat, rye, oats, corn/maize, malt, millet, barley, buck-wheat, cane sugar/syrup, grass and tree pollens	DAIRY PRODUCTS Cow's milk, cream, cheese, butter, yogurt, and products containing α-casein, beef, gelatin	EGGS All	YEAST Baker's yeast, brewer's yeast, yeast fractions as in wine, vinegar, bread, mushrooms, walnuts and molds
DAMAGING FRACTIONS	Gluten, α-gliadin and other glyco-protein fractions in wheat/grains; glycoprotein fractions in sugar, and glycoproteins in grass and tree pollens	Especially α-casein, α-lactalbumin, and β-lacto-globulin and beef albumin and globulin	Ovalbumin and egg globulins	Glycoprotein fractions of yeast, molds and virus capsules (Cf. GP 70 in capsule in Type cRNA viruses in murine SLE

OTHER FOODS CONTRAINDICATED IN SLE:

Curry, chili, sauces, spices, herbs, seasonings (contains pressor amines and vasoactive peptides that dilate capillaries, increasing permeability of toxic fractions, etc.)

Food additives, artificial colorings and preservatives (as well as certain drugs, estrogens, offending petrochemicals, etc., and too much sunlight)

ADDITIONAL FOODS FREQUENTLY OBSERVED TO AGGRAVATE SLE (IN OVER 600 CASES):

Onions, garlic, asparagus, ginger, peppers, capsicums, eggplant, paprika, choko, zucchini, mustard, small bananas, olives, chocolate, peanuts, pistachios, cinnamon, nutmeg, cola, licorice, oregano, sage, cloves, poppy seeds and specific food allergies/intolerances.
Foods to be limited to 2–3 times weekly:
    *Citrus, *tomatoes, cucumber, avocado
    *Totally avoid if antibodies to R.A. Latex, Rose Waaler, Synovial Membrane or Rheumatoid Factor are positive.

B. SAFER FOODS FOR SLE PATIENTS - PROVIDED NOT ALLERGIC/SENSITIVE FOLLOWING R.A.S.T., CYTOTOXIC, PROVOCATIVE OR CHALLENGE TESTS

The following foods should be safer:

GRAINS: Rice, sunflower seeds, sesame seeds; for bread/pastry – rice flour, arrowroot flour, potato flour, sweet potato flour, tapioca flour, sago flour

MILKS AND SUBSTITUTES: Goat's milk (not cheese or yogurt); for a baby, human milk with mother off cow's milk/gluten/other food allergies, coconut milk, agar instead of gelatin

MEATS: Chicken (unseasoned), turkey, duck, goose, pheasant, lamb, pork, rabbit, goat, deer

FISH: Especially sardines, pilchards, whiting, mackerel, salmon, bream, jewfish, kingfish, flounder, tuna, trout, snapper, flathead, etc., oysters, crab, squid, calamari (octopus), lobster, shrimp, scallops

NUTS: Cashews, almonds, hazelnuts, macadamias, brazilnuts, pecans, coconut

VEGETABLES: Tomato (twice weekly), potato, sweet potato, strawberries, cabbage, cauliflower, broccoli, brussel sprouts, dill, carrots, pumpkin, celery, cucumber (2–3 times weekly), spinach, watermelon, radish, watercress, rockmelon, parsnips, lettuce, beets, citrus

FRUITS AND BERRIES: Citrus occasionally – oranges, lemons, grapefruit, mandarins, tangerines, limes; grapes (washed), raspberries, blackberries, mulberries, loganberries, gooseberries, red currants, avocado (occassion-ally) pineapple, apricots, peaches, persimmon, lychees, blackcurrants, mango, pawpaw, apple (peeled), pear, custard apple, quince, passion-fruit, kiwifruit, big bananas, plums/prunes, figs (occassionally), dates (occassionally)

MISCELLANEOUS: Tea, maple syrup, parsley, safflower

Cytotoxic test results have served as useful pointers to other problem foods, many of which would not have otherwise been suspected. Cytotoxic positive foods, whose relevance is confirmed by symptom provocation on challenge after avoidance, are further avoided, but can sometimes be reintroduced in moderation after several months avoidance.

APPENDIX K

Avoiding a wheelchair

Help for your joints, skin, vessels and tissues

A. FOODS TO AVOID WITH SYNOVITIS/RHEUMATOID ARTHRITIS/VASCULITIS

Also helps patients with scleroderma, psoriatic arthritis, ankylosing spondylitis, Sjogren's Syndrome, primary biliary cirrhosis, schizophrenia, manic-depressive illness, OCD (obsessive-compulsive disorder), ADD (attention deficit disorder), hyperactivity, learning/behavior, sleep disorder, Gilles de la Tourette Syndrome, asthma and autism.

The foods to avoid are:

	GRAINS	DAIRY PRODUCTS	EGGS	YEAST
	Wheat, rye, oats, corn/maize, malt, millet, barley, buckwheat, cane sugar/syrup, grass and tree pollens	Cow's milk, cream, cheese, butter, yogurt, etc.; products containing α-casein; beef and gelatin	All	Brewer's yeast, baker's yeast and yeast fractions as in wine, vinegar, bread, mushrooms, walnuts and molds
DAMAGING FRACTIONS	Gluten and α-gliadin and other glycoprotein fractions in wheat/grains; glycoprotein fractions in sugar and glycoproteins in grass and tree pollens	Especially α-casein, α-lactalbumin and β-lactoglobulin and beef albumin and globulin	Ovalbumin and egg globulins	Glycoprotein fractions of yeast, molds and virus capsules. (Cf. GP70 in capsule in Type cRNA viruses in murine SLE

ALSO AVOID:

Cucumber, grapes, tea, citrus, legumes, beans, apples, almonds, plums/
prunes, strawberries, nectarines, passionfruit and kiwifruit

AVOID SOLANACEAE:

Potatoes, tomatoes, eggplant and capsicum

OTHER FOODS CONTRAINDICATED:

Curry, chili, sauces, spices, herbs, seasonings (contains pressor amines
and vasoactive peptides that dilate capillaries, increasing permeability
of toxic fractions, etc.)

Food additives, artificial colorings, preservatives (as well as certain drugs,
estrogens, offending petrochemicals, etc., and too much sunlight)

FOODS ALSO FREQUENTLY OBSERVED TO AGGRAVATE:

Onions, garlic, asparagus, ginger, peppers, capsicums, eggplant,
paprika, chokos, zucchini, mustard, small bananas, olives, chocolate,
peanuts, walnuts, pistachios, cinnamon, nutmeg, cola, kidney beans,
mung beans, licorice, oregano, sage, cloves, poppy seeds, and specific
food allergies/intolerances; rarely broccoli

B. SAFER FOODS (PROVIDED NOT ALLERGIC/SENSITIVE FOLLOWING RAST, CYTOTOXIC, PROVOCATIVE OR CHALLENGE TESTS).

GRAINS: Rice, sunflower seeds, sesame seeds and linseed; for bread,
pastry: rice flour, arrowroot flour, sweet potato flour, tapioca flour,
sago flour

MILKS AND SUBSTITUTES: Goat's milk (not cheese or yogurt); for a baby,
human milk with mother off cow's milk/gluten and other food allergies; coconut milk; agar instead of gelatin

MEATS: Chicken (unseasoned), turkey, duck, goose, pheasant, lamb,
pork, rabbit, goat, deer

FISH: Especially sardines, pilchards, whiting, mackerel, salmon, bream,
jewfish, kingfish, flounder, tuna, trout, snapper, flathead, etc., oysters,
crab, squid, calamari (octopus), lobster, shrimp, scallops

NUTS: Cashews, hazelnuts, macadamias, brazil nuts, pecans, coconut

VEGETABLES: Sweet potato, cabbage, cauliflower, broccoli, brussel
sprouts, dill, carrots, pumpkin, celery, radish, watercress, parsnips,
lettuce, beets, rockmelon and watermelon

FRUITS AND BERRIES: Raspberries, blackberries, mulberries, loganberries, red currants, avocado (occasionally), tinned pineapple, tinned apricots, tinned peaches, persimmon, lychees, blackcurrants, pawpaw, mango, pear, custard apple, big bananas, figs (occassionally), dates (occassionaly)

MISCELLANEOUS: Maple syrup (true), honey (not molasses honey), parsley, safflower, chamomile and dandelion tea

Cytotoxic test results have served as useful pointers to other problem foods, many of which would not have otherwise been suspected. Cytotoxic positive foods, whose relevance is confirmed by symptoms provocation on challenge after avoidance, are further avoided, but can sometimes be reintroduced in moderation after several months avoidance

REFERENCES

1. Woodward, R.J. and Blau, C.A. "Allergy testing." *Lancet,* 24 July 1987, p. 277.

2. Reading, C.M. Report for N.S.W. Cancer Council for year ended 30.6.1974, 89:37.

3. Reading, C.M. "Latent Pernicious Anaemia." *Med. J. Aust.,* 1(1975):430.

4. Reading, C.M. "Latent Pernicious Anaemia." *Med. J. Aust.,* 2(1975):111.

5. Reading, C.M. "Psychosurgery, Orthomolecular Psychiatry and the Press." *Med. J. Aust.,* 1(1977):642

6. Reading, C.M. "Down's Syndrome, leukaemia and maternal thiamine deficiency. *Med. J. Aust.,* 12(1976):505.

7. Reading, C.M., McLeay, A.C., Nobile, S. "Down's Syndrome and Thiamine Deficiency." *J. Orthomolecular Psychiatry*, 8(1979):1,4–12.

8. Reading, C.M. "X-linked dominant manic depressive illness: Linkage with Xg blood group, red-green colour blindness and vitamin B_{12} deficiency." *J. Orthomolecular Psychiatry.,* 8(1979):2, 68–77.

9. Reading, C.M. "Orthomolecular Psychiatry." *Med. J. Aust.,* 2(1979):40.

10. Reading, C.M. "Multiple Sclerosis: Is it transplacently induced?" *Med. Hypothesis,* 5(1979):11, 1251–1255.

11. Reading, C.M. "Klinefelter's Syndrome and biotin deficiency." *Med. Hypothesis,* 7(1981):1105–1108.

12. Reading, C.M. Address on Orthomolecular Medicine/Psychiatry to Medical Benefits Schedule Revision Committee, Dec. 3, 1980. Printed in *J. Orthomolecular Psychiatry,* 10(1981):1 29–34.

13. Reading, C.M. "Trace element metabolism on man and animal." *Discussions In* (J. Howell, J. Gawthorn, C.L. White); Canberra Austr.: Academy of Science, 1981.

14. Reading, C.M. "Relevance of cytotoxic test to detect food allergies/intolerance/hypersensitivity in psychiatric patients." Schizophrenia Assoc. of Great Britain Conference 22.4.1982, "Recent Trends in Biological Psychiatry."

15. Reading, C.M. Letter to Editor. *J. Orthomolecular Psychiatry,* 11(1982):2, 111–115.

16. Reading, C.M. Letter to Editor, *J. Orthomolecular Psychiatry* 11(1982):4, 276.

17. Reading, C.M. "Systemic Lupus Erythematosus: Nutritional Intervention." Address to 13th Annual Conference, McCarrison Society 23.8.1983. *Nutrition and Mental Health*: *Links between food and behaviour,* 1983.

18. Reading, C.M. "Down's Syndrome: Nutritional Intervention." Address to 13th Annual Conference, McCarrison Society, 23.8.1983, *Nutrition and Mental Health,* 3(1984):90–111.

19. Reading, C.M. "Down's Syndrome: Is gluten/alpha-gliadin sensitivity/coeliac disease the cause." *J. Biosocial Research,* 6(1984):62–65.

20. Reading, C.M. "Orthomolecular Psychiatry/Medicine." *Med. J. Aust.,* 1(1984):746.

21. Meillon, R.S., and Reading, C.M. *Relatively Speaking; Family Tree Way to Better Health.* Fontana Australia, Sydney, N.S.W. Australia, 1984.

22. Cooke, H.M. and Reading, C.M. "Dietary Intervention in Systemic Lupus Erythematosus: 4 cases of clinical remission and reversal of abnormal pathology." *International Clinical Nutrition Review,* 5(1985):4, 166–176.

23. Reading, C.M. "Dietary Intervention in Down's Syndrome: and a unifying theory as to its causation, prevention and treatment." Address to Annual General Meeting of Down's Syndrome Association of Queensland, 26.3.1986.

24. Reading, C.M. "Orthomolecular Genetics/ Medical Genealogy." Address to Australasian College of Biomedical Scientists, Leura, N.S.W., 20.9.1986.

25. Reading, C.M. "The Struggle for Acceptance of Biological and Molecular Psychiatry." *J. Australasian College of Nutritional and Environmental Medicine,* Oct. 1990, pp. 17–24.

26. Reading, C.M. "Nutritional Intervention for AIDS Patients." *J. Nutritional Medicine.,* 3(1992): 145–148.

27. Reading, C.M. "Advances in Orthomolecular Psychiatry." *Hypoglycaemia Health.* (March 1997), 13:1, 2–5.

28. Reading, C.M. "Is MS transplacentally induced?" *J. Australasian College of Nutritional and Environmental Medicine.,* Dec. 1997; pp. 18 and 24.

29. Reading, C.M. "Motor Neurone Disease and the Life of Motor Neurones. Is low B3/pellagra aggravating it?" *J. Australasian College of Nutritional and Environmental Medicine,* Dec. 1997, p. 21.

30. Reading, C.M. "Orthomolecular Psychiatry." *J. Australasian College of Nutritional and Environmental Medicine,* June 1998, p. 31.

INDEX

Ulcerative colitis, 69, 80, 243, 259, 261
Ulcers, 243–245, 249
Urticaria (hives), 69, 82–83, 124

Varicose veins, 33, 69, 152
Venous thromboses, 159
Villous atrophy, 241
Viral infections, recurrent, 124, 131, 139, 145, 147, 166, 172, 225
Vitamin(s)
    B family, 59, 150, 255–258, 261
    Biotin (Vitamin H), 255–258
    B_1, 47, 150, 203, 205, 207, 218, 230–231, 238, 246–247, 250–251, 255–258, 261
    B_3 (niacin), 47, 68, 70, 89, 150, 161-163, 200, 203, 205–206, 230–231, 238, 255, 261
    B_6, 41, 68, 70, 89, 110, 161–163, 167, 177, 205–206, 218, 230–231, 238, 247, 250, 255–258, 261
    B_{12}, 34–35, 47, 51, 54, 70, 72–73, 89, 112, 150, 154, 203, 237–238, 244–245, 259, 261
    C, 59, 118, 161–163, 184, 205–206, 218, 255–256
    E, 161–163, 218, 226

Vitiligo, 33–34, 79, 104–105, 199, 227, 246
Von Recklinghausen's Syndrome (neurofibromatosis), 113, 135

Werner's Syndrome, 136
Wilm's tumor, 133
Wilson's disease, 183
Wiskott-Aldrich Syndrome, 136–137

X chromosomes, 9, 23–29, 39–40, 51, 72, 84, 87–89, 107, 255
X-linked conditions, 23–28, 39–40, 43, 51, 53–55, 83, 85, 87, 89, 99, 101, 106–107, 134–137, 145, 173, 175, 182–183, 186, 209, 218, 223–224, 226, 237
Xerodoma pigmentosum, 133

Y chromosomes, 9, 23–29, 88
Y-linked conditions, 28–29, 42–45, 53–54

Zinc, 41, 120, 150, 162–163, 177, 184, 203, 205–206, 230, 255–256